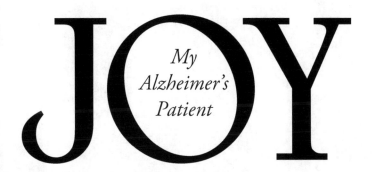

JOY

*My
Alzheimer's
Patient*

BRIGITTA HURD

BALBOA.
PRESS

A DIVISION OF HAY HOUSE

Balboa Press books may be ordered through booksellers or by contacting:

Balboa Press
A Division of Hay House
1663 Liberty Drive
Bloomington, IN 47403
www.balboapress.com
1 (877) 407-4847

Print information available on the last page.

ISBN: 978-1-5043-7947-2 (sc)
ISBN: 978-1-5043-7948-9 (e)

Balboa Press rev. date: 07/07/2017

CONTENTS

DEDICATION

This book is dedicated to the
teachings of Science of Mind
And to my Grandchildren
Camille, William, Bella, Ava and Gabriel,
Who opened my eyes to a World of Wonder.

Also included are my two older Grandsons Max
and Zac, who have managed to be instrumental
in the formulation of my ever expanding mind.

I would like to thank in spirit my dear friend
and editor Elizabeth Roberts, who was so
committed to this project, but had to follow the
call to a higher dimension.

To my sister Susanna and my dear friend Leni
Leth, who kept moving me forward and never
gave up, even when it looked like I did.

PROLOGUE

What am I going to do?
I don't want to be here.
I feel sick inside.
I am so unfulfilled.
It is almost like a depression.
Somebody help me!

All those thoughts and feelings are swirling through my head and mind. My legs are week and my fingers do not care to move. I sit down, close my eyes and start to breathe deeply. What have I learned all those years to come to such a low point in my life?

"Meditate," a bell is ringing from deep within, but loud enough to get my attention. Ah yes. *'Have you forgotten to still your mind and breathe deeply,'* the little voice reminds me? I feel better immediately. Time to ask for more direction and guidance. *'What am I to do with a job that pays well and gives me nothing?' I feel robbed and depleted of all my good energy.*

Answer number ONE

'Be the best you can be.' There it is. If I make the decision to stay on, I have to give the best of me at all times.

Clarity. The answer did not hit me like a lightning bolt, but rather folded over and around me like a preheated blanket. Warmth. I get it. Yes, yes, and yes again. I have to demonstrate the best of me. Why else would one perform a duty any other way?

More Meditation and more questions.

Answer number TWO:

"Journal," just like that. Journaling does not agree with me. Not that I don't realize the energy and power through the act of writing down what is in my head — it is just not my genre. Final answer.

"Journal," this little, ever so persistent voice insists and reminds me daily, hourly — no, constantly.

The minute I give my internal dialogue a break, "Journal" pops up without interruption. "But why should I journal and write down those boring hours of my work, especially when I don't find fulfillment in what I do?"

All right, I give up. I am going to do it. I will start journaling.

A few weeks go by since my first encounter with this voice from within. From now on I place every action I perform in the highest regard. I immediately elevate myself onto a higher pedestal and feel grand. Making a decision to better my actions, and therefore my life, almost gives me a jolt. Yes, that is the way life needs to be lived anyway — onward to a fabulous day.

CHAPTER ONE

My Time with an Alzheimer Patient

Spring 2011

I decided to start journaling the work I have been performing for the last four years — caring for an Alzheimer's disease patient, a field of service few of us really know much about.

Actually, the lady in my documentation is a distant in-law. Although not really in my field of employment, circumstances dictated that I start caring for Joy one day a week.

We always have a good time together. She loves to be driven or, as she calls it, "going for a ride."

By the time I arrive at her house in the morning, she greets me at the front door with a radiant smile. She is completely put together, including earrings, a scarf, a belt, lipstick and perfume, plus her beautifully tailored attire always matches from head to toe. Her hair is silver gray and cut in a pageboy style — beautiful! Joy is of slight build, a size eight, I would say, has a tiny waistline, and is about five foot, four inches tall.

We often drive all day long. I discover my new surroundings very quickly for it seems to me that driving Madame all over the place is all she cares about. Off we go, taking every major road, highway, and parkway so I can get it in my head how this unfamiliar landscape connects. Actually, it's like a joy ride. As a Southern California Girl transplant, now able to discover these spectacular neighborhoods in one of the most beautiful places in the world to live, it affords me a great opportunity.

We make excursions as far away as Laguna Beach, my mother's most favorite lunch destination. Whenever she visited from the old country, we both knew just where to go. Visiting this area of Southern California for a day with friends or family not only included lunch, but ocean views, spectacular vistas, and shopping. This is greatly differed from a gray November sky in Germany.

Joy's inner signal never fails to find a reason to

take a break. Hunger isn't it either, but the idea of a cocktail looming in the near future activates and mobilizes her thought process. She lets me choose the location of any restaurant, regardless of ethnic flavors. I just have to make sure cocktails are being served and a drink can be at hand. Getting stuck with just a glass of wine creates a huge shock to Joy's 'demanding' mind. It hasn't taken me very long to figure out how she lines up her priorities. A cocktail for lunch is a must and ordered before we even sit down. I cannot tell you how often we were just seated at our table and shortly after, her drink appears.

"Who ordered this?" I inquire.

You can guess the answer. Gin and tonic over ice with lime in a wine glass and a straw is standard. I opt for a glass of wine with soda for not having anything alcoholic to drink is unacceptable. When the bill arrives with a displeasing total, which they usually all do, she musters a look of disgust at me.

I start thinking, and don't ask me why, "*ashes to ashes, dust to dust,*" and then, of course, I burst out laughing at my ridiculous internal dialogue until Joy joins in.

Other times are not so smooth. We enter a

restaurant and Madame walks right by the hostess as though she owns the establishment, picks the best table by a window, and sits down. Reserved or not, it is now hers. First the hostess appears, informing us in a rather undiplomatic way that we can't just walk in and take over. To me, the situation becomes comical for the hostess does not have a clue as to whom she is dealing with. Joy is ready for WW III. Now the manager approaches. Of course, Madame may stay seated if she will please just calm down, curtail her terrible temper and stop screaming! I have to admit it is ugly.

After that particular scenario, I look at her and ask, as though I have been watching a performance, "Have you finished? Is that it?"

Joy looks straight at me, stunned. Then she studies me for a moment, glares past my face and up the walls to the ceiling, then down to her still empty plate.

"I'm ready for my cocktail and lunch."

Voila!

Suddenly, Joy starts telling me that she had been a good customer of the establishment and many others in the area, which should give her the right to sit anywhere she wants, especially if there is not a reserved sign visible. And so it is.

When I take over the position of Joy's regular companion and helper, I have no idea what I am getting into. It is her way or the highway, which involves yelling and getting physical. Nothing is ever good enough. The word "please" is not in her vocabulary; rather, not in her conscience. There are moments when she becomes so patronizing that I literally demand a "please" in order for me to do whatever she wants.

Her facial expression becomes almost wondrous, not understanding, it appears, why the word is necessary or why she needs to utter it in order to get her demands fulfilled. The tantrums must have worked for Joy all of her life. I truly believe that she frightened everyone around her with her rather ugly way of screaming. She had used it to always get her way. Unfortunately, her friends, family, and whoever she came in contact with had not been taught about detachment.

Too late for me to think I can make a difference, especially since she is disinterested. After all, I am dealing with a woman who has been diagnosed with Alzheimer's disease. I am accustomed to entertaining the thought of change.

It is important for me to take the time to contemplate our daily activities and thought processes. It is so easy to get off track. Every day is the same scenario:

Close that door.

Close that window.

Cover the butter.

Put that here.

Get the shoes.

Hang this up.

Let's go for a ride down the highway.

The good part is that I already know that she does not mean any harm or intends to create a dim atmosphere.

She has an innocent way of apologizing, "Did I offend you?"

Or she mentions that she really did not mean it at all and I should ignore that part. Then we laugh at each other and all is forgotten.

Being able to detach myself from this constant banality lightens the baggage — baggage that most of us seem to carry. No matter what is said, I will not let it faze me for I know that it simply has nothing to do with me.

Our dynamics work so well that within a few months we cease to have disagreements or arguments. The other caretakers constantly complain about her and literally beg me to order some tranquilizers from her physician. I did and must admit that I was horrified when I read about the side effects. Her doctor explained to me that the drug is commonly used. The decision is between my conscience and the medicine. I just cannot do it, especially when realizing that only the other caregivers have difficulties keeping Joy at bay. They need to be trained to detach themselves or maybe *they* need to be medicated!

Always having had domestic help or someone working for her keeps Joy in a demanding mode at all times. I was warned that I might not be able to handle her. I just smiled at the time for I knew I could.

One thing I have learned — now I know for sure that I can handle anyone who crosses my path. I might not like or enjoy their company, but whatever time we spend together will be peaceful.

Get on the wagon and detach from the outcome — "the magic lies in the details."

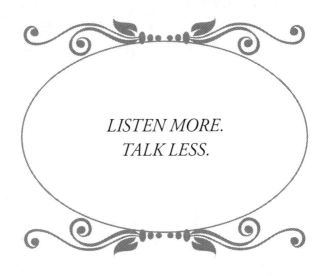

LISTEN MORE.
TALK LESS.

Chapter Two

Joy, My Alzheimer Patient

Joy is changing again. She no longer registers the seasons with their magic. She barely lifts her eyes towards the door to greet a visitor. Her eyes are fixed on the TV, or maybe she stares right through the monitor? No, none of the above. Her eyes are open and her 'being' seems to be inward only. She doesn't have a clue as to what is going on in her house.

Telephone, television, conversations between others — it is all gone. She still can fake it a bit when she experiences an 'aha' moment. Then she remembers a 'mechanical' answer from her memory bank. Joy takes much longer now to complete her mealtime and is eating considerably less. Just when I decide that nothing mattes to her, it does.

Fast food establishments, including their

contents, are not part of Joy's makeup. I am delighted. We now go less often to a restaurant during my shifts, which make the occasional dinner excursion more special. If we end up dining just around the corner, I allow myself a cocktail. By the time we depart from the establishment, an hour and a half has gone by, which in my mind makes it responsible enough. I always have to feel good making the decision, being aware of the circumstances.

During our time getting ready, we usually start by Joy brushing her teeth. I turn around for a moment, giving her enough time to take the toothbrush with the toothpaste and rub it into her hair. Detecting turquoise paste on her silver-white crown, Joy is faster than I am, grabs her hairbrush and proceeds with gentle strokes, maybe deciding she is able to get it out. Or maybe she likes the aqua color on her now beautiful white hair and delights in brushing the paste in.

No matter what I say or do, a reaction hardly follows. Questioning her does not help the matter for she mostly closes her eyes. I am on my own.

Routines are boring, no doubt, no matter how many people feel the contrary. I also do not believe an Alzheimer's patient needs a routine, especially if they are the ones who are unable to remember what happened a few minutes ago. Nevertheless, I am learning as I go and might change my mind. There are other caregivers and one, in particular, is all about routine.

"Joy needs to have her routine."

I get it now. It's all about the caregiver's preference for routine.

Joy goes with the flow and takes plenty of opportunities to let me know that she is glad to be with me. I may take her anywhere my heart desires and drive as far as I wish for she will delight in it. How about that? Time is of no essence. I am ready to think of a place to stop for dinner when she suggests a drive to San Diego.

Any personal hygiene by Joy is now extinct. Once in a while, she appears in the morning with her hair brushed and lipstick on. How is it possible that she looks so radiant just like that? Her appearance is also my reminder to get ready to leave the house.

It takes longer for my beauty treatment. Straight out of bed I look terrible in the morning and no matter in which direction I turn, a huge mirror stares me in the eyes. No chance to ignore this kind of 'wall.'

The only one besides Joy who has the pleasure of seeing me au natural is my husband of almost forty-five years. He still insists that I look beautiful without any makeup. What a man! I look in the mirror again and wonder what he sees. I must confess, I appreciate those comments more and more. We had a lot of fun together, but we also had our rocky roads. Nevertheless, he is the kind of man one wants to end up with.

Younger women take longer to apply all available makeup. Hair extensions, wigs, fake eyelashes, push-up bras, body enhancers, spandex, butt lifters, and who knows what all is available these days to look more and more perfect and fantastic — not to forget membership in a gym or yoga class. If you are not jumping or at least being physically active, what's wrong with you?

Don't forget that we need classes for our Soul. In the advanced stage of life, the inner beauty expresses itself as much as we let it. It happens through living a more balanced life, taking deeper breaths, giving love and kindness more readily, experiencing joy in our daily lives, and hopefully applying and acting on the lessons learned throughout time.

Joy's incontinence is present, but only to the extent of two maxi diapers in twenty-four hours. She still goes to the bathroom by herself and has not had any bad accidents, thank goodness. Then it happens and it is awful. There is a saying, "What does not kill you makes you stronger," and it does. I shared my plight with a nurse who mentioned that calcium could be a culprit for disaster. Sure enough, I had just purchased one of the better brands, a potent calcium. Suggested dosage: two capsules.

Days must seem ephemeral to Joy for they go on and on with not much in between. At times, she exhales so vocally I believe something is stirring in her mind.

Yesterday, she stays in bed all day. We have a good breakfast together. After completion, Joy vanishes into her bedroom and remains there until about four PM. Three times during the day I go in and ask her to join me for lunch. I even open her covers for an easier exit. Nothing happens. She is all wrapped up like a sushi roll and not approachable. During one of my returns, I gesture towards the highway, hoping to excite her about an upcoming ride. Nothing. She goes to the bathroom and back to bed.

I think, why not? She certainly has earned the right to stay in bed once in a while and if it makes her feel good, by all means. How wonderful that Joy has the privilege of remaining in the comfort of her home.

I used to volunteer at a skilled nursing facility. The attendants were very nice and caring, but had to stick to a strict routine, not always in favor of their patients. Being attentive during that time opened my eyes and heart to all people and personnel who give of their time, patience, and love on a daily basis.

I have made it clear to my children that they should never worry about me. If I cannot take care of myself and have become senile, put me in a home. How can I feel this way?

For 'now' is the best of times.
The best is here.
The best has arrived.
The best is at your front door.
The best of times are now.

We have forgotten to look for the best. We have neglected the desire to find the best.

I had questioned my Mom about the best times of her life when she came over to live in the United States. She was seventy-two years of age. (I am almost there!)

She answered, "Now Gittelein [her endearing name for me]," her eyes ablaze, "Now is the time for we have the present moment."

She was always so right on. The more mature I become, the more I admire her.

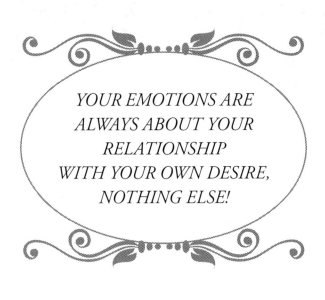

*YOUR EMOTIONS ARE
ALWAYS ABOUT YOUR
RELATIONSHIP
WITH YOUR OWN DESIRE,
NOTHING ELSE!*

CHAPTER THREE

What is Happening to My Patient?

Yes, I am still with Joy. The weeks and months have gone by and the changes are very subtle but every bit worth reporting.

While the routine of the day does not change, her attention span has. The TV has completely lost its lure. The only time I turn it on is strictly for my entertainment while being active in the kitchen or taking care of Joy. I experience fleeting moments visualizing her losing it completely in any way that you chose to interpret this.

It happened just a few days ago. I am quite amazed about myself at how I handled this for I made up my mind ages ago never to go this far. I know I am able and can do anything that comes my way for I have learned through my life experiences.

Joy walks into the kitchen surrounded by

an odor reserved for your imagination and beyond description. I am able to stop her from sitting down just in time. With a bit of finesse, concentrating on keeping my mouth shut (it is tempting to mumble, grumble or scream), I coax her into an 180° turn around. In the bathroom, I quickly grab and slide on latex gloves, strip her of every stitch of clothing and into the shower she goes. She sees what happened and literally does not understand the situation. Joy washes without soap. It is now up to me to enter the rather large shower as well. She is able to sit down and with the shower gel in hand, I undertake the mission of making sure she smells clean as a powder puff.

When everything is over and Joy is cleaned up, the soiled clothing washing away in top-notch appliances, the walker cleaned and sanitized, the toilette scrubbed inside and out, and her bed freshly changed, I sit down with her and give thanks internally to whoever was listening, for now I know I can do anything.

Anyone in the medical field might think, "Oh brother, what's the big deal?" True. If you have chosen to become a nurse or a caregiver, I believe this is your profession and you execute the duties that fall under those categories.

My vocation was in the hospitality field, not hospital. I imagine most of my readers are mothers, fathers, wives, husbands, partners, sons, daughters, companions, or grandparents. It looks like everyone is covered but children.

The good thing is that Joy shows willingness to do whatever I direct her to do as I gesture and give her physical assistance, of course. Lots of plastic bags are a must to help in the control of the ghastly emitter in my hands. Never did I contemplate working to this point of my patient's condition, but amazingly enough, here I am and still alive.

I learned years ago that I am able to do anything I put my mind to. Therefore, my actions depend on my willingness to do them. My mind says, "No, I don't want to do this," while my subconscious moves me forward with, "Of course I can." We know by now that the subconscious always wins. It is up to you now to research this phenomenon. The more you actively do the things you did not think you could do, the more powerful you will feel and become. It almost feels as though you are floating on a magic carpet. A feeling of fearlessness enters your being, culminating in your detachment.

You have arrived at a meaningful stage of your life. What a sense of accomplishment. Congratulate yourself. Be proud and always carry your head high. We are not talking about aloofness; no, just a knowing smile on your face, a wink of your eye, and a feeling of pleasure spreading its wings all over you.

Yesterday, we started a reality show, episode one, and, as we know, there is more to come.

My little granddaughter Bella is waiting for us at my house to be picked up and spend the night with Joy and me. This girl is so highly spirited and entertaining that we love being in her company. We have some great laughs together while the change of tapestry during Easter vacation benefits young and old.

The evening starts off rather smoothly with Joy constantly wondering who this girl is and why she is with us in the car. Driving down the coast, we slow down for a traffic check. Any time there is a slow-down or an out-of-control situation, Joy makes a conscious decision to go to the bathroom.

I make it clear to her that there are no accommodations in our direction. That goes on for a while, but she just does not want to accept my story.

"They should have a toilet," she keeps saying to herself over and over.

Once the traffic starts moving again, not another word is mentioned on the subject.

Finally, we arrive at our destination, one of our favorite restaurants.

Whenever we have company for dinner, which means someone else besides Joy and me, she decides not to be hungry. She does not want to order at all or will choose the least expensive item on the menu. She becomes extremely concerned that she does not have enough money to take care of the bill.

I order a scampi appetizer for Joy and also for my grandchild. Joy cannot get over the price and keeps saying (nine times, at least) how reasonable our dinner is. Obviously, she looked at the appetizer prices compared to the dinner menu. Enough said for she still only eats her roll with a load of butter and a few bites of the rest.

The time comes for our departure. Joy grabs the two 'to-go-bags,' which are overloaded to begin with, plus reaches for her purse while I am busy trying to drape her long coat over her shoulders. She is so determined to control the situation that any kind of interference is a hindrance to her. All this happens within seconds for Joy is completely obsessed with hanging on to her purse and in fear of us forgetting the packaged leftovers. She puts everything in one hand and with the other reaches to fetch her purse and grab the walker. Unbelievable.

Normally, all of the ballast would be hanging on me but not tonight. Madame has the urge to take charge and do whatever she can. The customers close by stare at her, then at my grandchild and me and back to Joy, trying to figure out if we are family and, I am quite sure, why I am not helping this poor (but stubborn) woman as we proceed towards the exit.

Oops! Her purse flips open, the 'to-go' falls on the floor and the grandchild at the tail end plays Hansel and Gretel, searching for all the lost items. What a show. I just have to let her do this for observing our show does end up with a good laugh, including Joy. It is amazing how her psyche is still influenced by her immediate surroundings. What she ignores at home becomes a completely different scenario when we are in public.

I have listened to this ninety-nine times plus. Who knows? It may have been going on for years. My reply is just as repetitious for I feel this yearning of someday making a difference with her. It has not happened yet.

When she gets tired of hearing me express delight over the magnificent ocean views, sunsets, and diverse vistas, of talking about balance in ourselves and in our lives, she takes a deep breath and looks straight ahead, chin in the air. The message is clear.

Another day is a sleepy one. The sky along the ocean communities is gray and decides to stay that way all day. The message is clear: hang out at home and relax. In the afternoon, we take a long ride and come home to go to bed by nine o'clock in the evening. Joy goes 'out' like a light. Dinner is skipped. All is well.

The next day seems to be a lost one. There is absolutely no reaction to anything from the minute Joy gets up. A royal breakfast is served without any emotion on her part. It is difficult for me to watch this for 'food' is such a major part of my existence.

We go out to our favorite Thai dinner house. After our meal, Joy watches me pay the check with a credit card. Back in the car, she inquires about the dinner check and its amount. I tell her the amount was $30.00, plus $6.00 for the tip. Her mind is at work. She decided that she owes me $15.00, plus $3.00 for the gratuity, which totals $18.00. I am amazed. Now Joy fishes at her feet for her purse, which is in the back seat and absolutely not reachable. She works at it for at least 15 minutes, using her right arm, then the left, determined to grab her purse. Then she tries unsuccessfully to unbuckle herself. She is wearing a leather jacket, which obstructs her view of the buckle. Her mind does not let her rest and she goes through the whole financial scenario over and over again. By the time we arrive at home, my cut is down to $10.00. With zeal in mind, up the step she goes, into the laundry room and immediately searches her purse for cash. She grabs her wallet, retrieves a $5.00 bill, which she places on my handbag, and tells me she owes me another $5.00. I so love it when I see her still able to think.

By now, she is appalled at the dollar amount for our exceptionally delicious meal. A promise from me to not spend any money the next day for dinner makes her soften up a bit. We will stick to this and finish all leftovers for the next day's meal.

I enjoy just getting in the car and driving without having to get all dressed up for a big dinner ceremony. Crazy enough, it is my ceremony. Joy is the one who always looks so radiant. She also has elegance about her, enhanced by a beautiful wardrobe. I feel compelled to do as much as I can to be part of her appearance. In addition, Madame is twenty years older than I am and receives all the attention and smiles from onlookers.

This morning at an early breakfast, Joy decides that too much is going on in her house without her awareness. Assuring her that I always let her know if the carpet cleaner is on the way, the floor tiles need fixing, the stovetop has to be replaced, or the washer/dryer are in need of repair, seems to calm her down. By the time of the event, it is all forgotten and no matter how often I explain this to her, given the situation, she is not convinced at all. I avoid mentioning to Joy that in each case I have called and asked her son for permission. That does not sit well with her at all.

"I am the owner of this house and I make the decisions!"

"This is the reason we are with you, Joy, as you forget what happens around you and in your life. We are here to keep you safe and your household running smoothly," I explain.

Maybe the sentence is too long; even so, I stand

right in front of her and repeat my words. She has already decided against all this and answers right away with a long, "Noooo."

Joy goes back to bed and it is not a surprise when she picks up this train of thought after her nap. It can also go the other way: "What's going on here?" might come out of her mouth, or "Would you like to go for a ride?"

The shift of thought arrives slowly but apparent in the way she words her questions. "Let's go for a ride," is the bull's eye of her universe. There is no question about the internal feeling as to what her needs are at any moment in time. "Let's get ready and get out of here," is all that counts in her now limited existence.

Generally, I enter her room, open all the shades and windows, marvel aloud at the beautiful day outside, sing a song, and then proceed to her bedside to ask her to get up. Her look is blank and half-questioning as to what I say. "What do you want or mean?" I interpret her expression.

The minute I answer with, "Let's go for a ride," enforcing my suggestion with "down the boulevard," we are on.

She gets it and by mustering all her strength, she works herself out of bed.

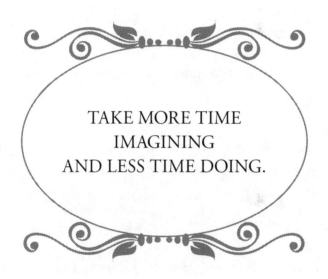

TAKE MORE TIME
IMAGINING
AND LESS TIME DOING.

CHAPTER FOUR

The Light at the End of the Tunnel

Worrying and getting involved in a thousand little chitchatting thoughts is a waste of energy.

"Let it be," is what I have gotten out of it for it does not matter anyway, or does it? I used to test myself by asking the same old questions: "What will I do if I only have a short while to live or I receive devastating news?"

What would I change? No reason to wait until this might happen. Now is the time. Don't sweat the small stuff. Look towards the light at the end of the tunnel.

Being diagnosed with Alzheimer's disease has to be devastating news. Nobody likes to hear this or can ever prepare oneself. By watching the public TV channel, I have learned that keeping our minds active and in a constant learning mode can literally prevent or slow down this condition. There is more to it but not in my capacity to discuss.

Joy still has this dazzling look and I know how important it is for her when someone recognizes her with a greeting or just a friendly smile. She has the ability to light up a room. How wonderful is that?

Gradually, ever so gradually, her Spirit is less and less noticeable. When her awareness returns, if only for a moment, her interlude is short and to the point. There is no doubt that she once was a smart businesswoman.

I have mentioned patience before and cannot stress enough how vital this is in caring for an Alzheimer's patient. The constant repetition of actions and monotonous verbal communications has been and are still very taxing to caregivers.

Joy can sit at the table, for example, and start burping and burping very loud, then yawning over and over again, adding to the pool of noises. One has the desire to scream, just that, scream as loud as possible. That part, thank goodness, has been lived and is passé.

Now is the time and opportunity to practice

what I have learned. What was that again? Patience. We have to practice patience.

Patience means taking a deep breath before proceeding. It has been said, in the context of changing the world, that a deep breath before we act instead of answering with a kneejerk reaction has the power to change the 'dynamics' or the 'vibrations' we emit as energy coming from the processing of our thoughts, which then, in turn, influences the outcome.

There is the light at the end of our famous tunnel. Now is the time. Don't sweat the small stuff.

If we are reflecting on the light at the end of the tunnel, we must not forget the acceptance. Acceptance is essential in order to see the light, in order to be joyful and feel happy. No way can we be critical or judgmental and expect a fulfilling and interesting life.

Accepting what is leads to my feelings of freedom, especially in situations I know I am not able to change. The sooner I let them go and concentrate on what I 'can' do or am able to change, the energy shifts towards a positive and satisfying outcome. Doors we have not imagined will open.

If we start looking at the little occurrences

in our lives, observing how fortunate we are to be able to set the dinner table with a cloth and napkins, decorate with flowers, add silverware, dishes, and drinking glasses all available to us, we have to start feeling grateful.

Now we add and serve FOOD for all in the family, plus friends. A splendor in varieties of meats and seafood, or produce, organic fruits and vegetables, herbs and spice, shipped and delivered to us from near and far and readied through our open market and grocery stores. As far as libations are concerned, the varieties are endless. No staying in long lines, having to fight for a loaf of bread or some protein. Everything imaginable is there for our choosing. We are so blessed. It is actually a miracle. Fifty years ago, one hundred years ago, this life of richness and diversity was unimaginable. Let us be grateful from morning to night. Be mindful of your thoughts and hidden desires. Make them come alive by believing you have received them already and watch what happens. Your experiences will be life changing.

Just keep saying "Thank you."

There is a light at the end of your tunnel.

We just have to learn to believe it, expect it, see it, and live as though it has already arrived.

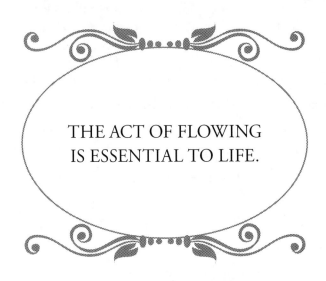

THE ACT OF FLOWING
IS ESSENTIAL TO LIFE.

CHAPTER FIVE

What is Going On?

We are the creators of harmony or dissent. This I can feel more each day for changes are happening, ever so subtly, but they are coming.

The whole household feels the subsiding energy. Or is it more a shift? Maybe Joy's energy stays inward and simply cannot escape her prison within.

I know we are vibrational beings. Consequently, I am reacting towards the energy Joy emits — energy, in my evaluation, so low that a feeling of nothing, a feeling of emptiness, an awareness of a house without air or oxygen or even life comes over me.

I wonder what she is feeling. What is left at this point?

As far as I am concerned, 'nothing' can be left up to her thought processes. Any question I pose is answered with a blank stare or the occasional closing of her eyes. Recognition is at its lowest point. No matter how much I point a direction with my finger, it is now completely ignored.

We return from dinner and a visit with Joy's new great-grand baby. She applied herself for a moment or two with the little one but mostly stared into space.

I drive daily along the ocean and its shores, only to realize with great sadness her inability to capture the beauty all around us. The magnificent sunset leaves her unmoved and motionless no matter how much I exclaim my excitement and wonder. Her eyes have lost their spark and she is unaware of the coming and going of humanity. What she does see, and will go to great acrobatic gestures to retrieve, are specks of paper on the floor or anything she just dropped, such as an earring or food, paper napkin or tissue.

However, her eyes are amazingly sharp for a woman of almost eighty-nine years of age. She does not miss the signs along the roadside nor the illumination as we drive into the night.

The day before, she noticed nothing to her left or right — just her tunnel vision. Now, part of the 'former' lady is back.

"Is it okay to read the signs out loud?" she keeps asking me while I drive.

I squeeze her arm gently and smile. Sometimes I rub her hands. At the beginning, she would just look at me and pull her hand away. Now, she has become the woman she really is beneath all the cover-up of our humanness. So we wonder; at least that is what I do.

It is the next day and time for our excursion. Let's get started. Before leaving the house, we freshen up.

Getting Joy out of bed gives me another strange feeling for she has no idea what the next step ahead has in store for her. I can read it from her wondering and perplexed expression.

I guide her and her supportive walker into the bathroom. The walker, by now, is Joy's rock, or so I thought until I left her in the car by herself. The only time I allow myself the luxury of doing some errands is after I take her to the bathroom and let her stay in the car to watch the traffic go by. She usually has to go between one and one-and-a-half hour increments. Joy does not like to get out of the car and will do anything she can to convince me of her dismay. I park in front of a drugstore behind a planted median, a location that is familiar to her.

Joy promises to stay put and to speed up the time of my absence, I take a shortcut through the little bushes and run into the building. Ten minutes these days is the maximum allowable point of testing her patience.

I make it my business to familiarize myself with all the stores I frequent so I know exactly which isle I can find what I need. If more time is needed, I take Joy with me. I know it is hard for her to move, but on the other hand, it is also important for her body to experience some activity. I often schmooze with her a bit by letting her know how much I like her input while shopping, which, indeed, is the truth for Madame has good taste.

Whether she likes it or not, slowly, and without giving me a long look that translates "all right, you got me," she will release her seatbelt and off we go.

So there she is in the car, nodding her head as a 'good bye,' making me feel a little more comfortable as I dash off. This time, I cannot find the items I need as fast as planned. By the time I step out of the store, I see Joy struggling to make her way through the bushes. She reaches for a parked basket, halfway hanging on, standing on a wobbly rock, and giving me 'the look': "I'm almost there. It's just a little more cumbersome then I anticipated."

No walker, no safety net. Oh my goodness! My brain spins in disbelief. It is good fortune that Joy is still in an upright position. Her walker is in the backseat of the car and therefore out of her sight and mind. Obviously, the time has come to make adjustments.

The next day we take off like always, cruising along the highway. I need an itinerary to keep my sanity. Just driving without a Ziel [destination] in mind is almost hypnotizing.

I take another chance. What is the definition of 'insanity' again? Doing the same things over and over and expecting different results.

Into the store I run, and out in exactly four minutes, just long enough to catch Joy already in the process of pushing the door open to step out.

"Joy, where are you going?" I call.

Her answer is clear. "I have to go to the bathroom."

"No you don't, Joy. We just went about ten minutes ago." This, of course, means nothing to her at all.

Back in the car, we just drive round the bend to the drugstore parking lot and she asks to go again. No matter the location we approach, I always look for bathroom signs and steer Joy in the other direction to avoid going into a stall every few minutes. The instant she discovers the handicap plaque, the 'W' or 'Women' signage on any building, it's over and we must use the facility.

At home, on the way to the garage and her car, we have to pass the guest bathroom, which she simply cannot and will not ignore, even after finishing on her own toilet a few minutes prior.

In Joy's bathroom, when I prepare the toothbrush with paste ready for her application, her look is blank. She waits for further instructions. I motion to her how to proceed and she copies me. Next is the washcloth. I start with cold water for her face, which she still manages to apply by herself and enjoys. I diligently wash her upper body. Depending on her mental outlook of the day, she volunteers for the job.

When the time comes to help Joy with her personal hygiene, she avoids the use of soap, which I find surprising, particularly knowing her to be quite the opposite.

I call a friend whose husband has Alzheimer's disease. It is the same situation. He does not want to be showered or bathed and will do anything to avoid the suds. How interesting is that? At least I now know this behavior is indicative of Alzheimer's disease.

I fill the sink full of warm water to take care of Joy's lower torso but not before Joy wipes the counter for the fourth or seventh time, either with a washcloth or over-used tissue. As far as Joy is concerned, it has to be done and I have grown to let it all happen the way her mind needs it to be. If we don't get in the way of ourselves, we achieve much more in peace and harmony.

With latex gloves on my hands, I soap up the washcloth for the lower part of her body. Most of the time I do the washing, front and back. Sometimes she reaches for the cloth to wash herself. At times, she makes it clear who is in charge. Unfortunately, I do have to intervene for Madame insists on proceeding without soap.

Baby powdered all around and with a fresh pull-up diaper, we move into the dressing stage and walk towards her bed. I select Joy's bra, blouse, long pants, socks and shoes and, after massaging her body and face with lotion — Joy manages to apply her deodorant — it is time to get dressed. Whatever her attire, the choice is now up to me. Draped with her clothing, I officially introduce myself as her personal dresser.

This day I am lucky. She smiles at my appearance, or maybe she is the lucky one for she must feel something. Back in the bathroom, I brush her beautiful silver-white hair and apply dark-colored lipstick, which looks striking with her complexion. Time for her earrings, scarf, or any selection from the array of accessories to adorn her beauty. Now Madame is ready and unstoppable.

Joy showers every other day. Five years ago, when I started caring for her, she refused to shower. With the support of her son, we tried everything, to no avail. In fact, she tricked me, going into the bathroom and closing the door right in my face — click. All right, I think, *do it yourself.*

Yeah, right. She turned the water on in the shower while dressing herself. When I finally opened the bathroom door, she pretended to be busy doing something else while standing there in her undies and the top of her pajamas. I stared at her in disbelief.

At the look on my face, she reacted by immediately exclaiming, "Oh yes, I showered."

The "avoid a shower under any circumstances" went on for almost a year and was over as suddenly as it started.

Off to the garage we march, through the kitchen, with a short stop at the bathroom, through the laundry room, then using the walker to get down one step and onto the seat of her automobile. There she sits, quite content, always expecting my instant appearance.

I take care of my face, clothes, and accessories as fast as I can to keep up with her tempo. Time for a change, which translates: time for me to change something. First and most important, I get completely ready before awakening Joy. Then I prepare a snack and arrange it on the kitchen table, the TV turned on.

When Joy approaches this area, she sees the lures, sits down, eats, and watches the TV screen, while I have the time for final touches. It is working perfectly!

Once Joy is situated in the car with her seatbelt on, I have a happy and content camper at my side.

CHAPTER SIX

Be the Change You Want to See

Being with my Alzheimer patient is life changing.

Driving to work in the morning with my window down is a joy to me. I cruise along the ocean, watching business people sweeping the sidewalks, early walkers and joggers, and sometimes I get lucky and smell fresh coffee and bacon. What a way to start the day.

Here is one side of the coin.

First choice: "I am dreading this day already."

It is the same day every day, void of conversation, but always having to say something. Joy expects it. Routine after routine, until I interrupt. The whole day is more or less programmed; so are the TVs in every room. Joy's personal noises are the worst and could drive one crazy.

Now, my second choice:

I am curious to see how Joy is today. I wonder about her. Bless her heart and her soul. She is trying so much to do what she still can comprehend and would like to accomplish. Indeed, at times she can and has a blissful moment. I have to pay attention and give her this understanding.

I hear her coming from the bedroom into the kitchen with her walker, her security. When I smile at her, she smiles back. She does not recognize me at this moment in time. When I forget to smile, she stares blankly. I help her into the chair and push her closer to the table. This is muscle work. She eats and stares. She watches TV and stares. She looks at me and through me. I am smiling. Her smile is blank. I am her family for the moment and for the moment that means her whole life.

Joy stares at the plate I set on the place mat and waits for me to sit down and start eating. She copies what I do. When she is hungry, she acts as if she is famished and attacks her food, especially a sandwich freshly grilled. This does not happen very often for Madame is not a 'foodie' as I am. I love my cooking and devour every bite. Frankly, watching me indulge puts a smile on her face.

Once in a while she even comments, "You do love to cook," and we lock eyes in harmony.

Time for myself — a nap.

Joy does not go into the kitchen to cook any more or to start up any appliances. There is a glass-top stove, which is foolproof and at this stage, invaluable. The house is surrounded by tall brick walls connected with iron gates, which are locked at all times. The only way out for her is through the house and into the garage. On the wall is the garage door opener. She still knows how to handle this button. I have snuck up behind her when I heard her walking away from our usual area in the kitchen. She stands at the driveway. Does she wonder at the smells in the air, or is she unable to figure out where she is anymore? She is wearing her pajamas for nothing mundane matters any more.

Time to get ready for the day. After she is washed and dressed, sitting on her bed, I leave her with three chores to do: apply lipstick, brush her hair, and put on earrings. Sometimes she has it altogether, other times she does not. Her lovely white hair shines brightly, her earrings give her sparkle, and her painted dark lips pronounce the beautiful woman she still is. We keep her perfume, a lipstick, a hairbrush, and another pair of earrings in her car, just in case.

Time to cruise up or down the coast. She loves it. Taking care of errands is no longer in the cards for Joy does not listen, or even understand what I tell her to do or not to do. If I step out of the car, even for just a short while, she might wonder where she is, feel lonely, get out and walk off. Running into the local cleaner still works. She likes to sit there in the hope that the owner will come out to say hello to her. Joy is always in the mood for a flirt. I still dare a quick run into the drugstore. Fast. Everything is timing.

Bombarding Joy with questions is agony for her. Alzheimer patients cannot formulate an answer and by making the effort to do so, time elapses and they forget what the question is about. That frustrates Joy very much, which she clearly expresses by getting irritated. This is a time for us caregivers to know her needs, likes, and dislikes. She is not a danger to herself, but if left alone in the house for the day, she would wander off. The minute it gets dark, she demands a person by her side. I do not know what this is within her, but her eyes are wide open and follow my every move.

Just hanging up her clothes and going in and out of her bedroom and bath makes her uneasy.

"What are you doing?"

"Are you coming into my room? (I am there.)

"Are you coming into my bed?"

"Where are you going?"

I play charades to let her know of my impending personal hygiene attempt. After about three minutes, I hear her come into my room. I used to get upset over this every night and tried to stop her from repeating the visits.

> We enter a New Year, an opportunity
> to drop old habits and start anew.

I have to be the change I want to see.

Now, when Joy appears at my door, which I keep open at all times, I invite her in to sit on my bed and wait for me. Sometimes she returns to her bed and sometimes she sits down and watches TV and me at the same time until I finish. Then, a month later, she stays in her bed and is quite content to wait for me.

Always those little things that have the ability, if we allow them, to cause us to act so poorly or foolishly.

CHAPTER SEVEN

The Subject Matter

Yes, I am taking care of an Alzheimer's patient. Yes, it is very testy at times and situations have a way of becoming quite difficult. Have there been missteps, accidents, and surprises? Indeed! Plenty of times.

Realizing that I exclude the unwanted from my consciousness (and am forever working on this), I shall summarize some experiences about my dealings with unusual situations.

Joy was once a strong-willed and strong-minded woman, also very disciplined and orderly. This was immediately apparent when entering her home. Anyone stepping into the house, even before given the chance of leaving the door open or ajar for more than a second, was told in a rather commanding way, "Close that door!"

She no longer registers open doors and

cabinets, even while sitting at the breakfast table, which is, to me, utterly amazing.

Yesterday we had a visitor and Joy immediately called out, "Close that door." We quietly giggled, for every door and cupboard was closed. The command came from Joy's mouth automatically.

At this point, every sentence Joy speaks comes from her sub-conscious mind. It just has to be that way for she is no longer able to formulate any present thought process (if there even is one) into a sentence. Any time she wants to say something, it turns into a mumble. Absolutely nothing comes out but a raspy rumble, which she quickly stops. I believe she has already lost track of her intention.

She does not seem that frustrated about this matter for I don't hear anything but a deep exhale. It feels more as if she is 'giving up' as she stares straight out of the window. On the other hand, what else can she do? Frustrated? Depressed?

What does she compute?

What does she understand?

How much of a conversation does she comprehend?

At this point, more than I realize. Somehow, I can feel it.

On a recent night, I drove quite a distance to

meet with my husband and an out-of-town friend for dinner. I have noticed before that when we meet with other people to dine, Joy barely touches her meal. She mostly opens the menu, glances at it, and then decides to split whatever I have. I always consult with her and then order.

Bread and butter are items she cannot resist. When the actual dinner arrives, right away she raises her voice with, "no, no, no," and pushes her plate away. This particular evening she repeats the same scenario.

Our friend had planned to invite us anyway and I assured Joy of this by whispering the good news into her ear. When all is done and paid, Joy tells me in a clear manner of her concern. She did not eat anything; therefore, my friend should have paid only for her drink.

What do we know? How will we ever know what goes on in her head at this time and in her condition?

A typical morning with Joy begins when I go into her room between nine and ten to wake her up and ask her to join me for breakfast. She has no clue any more as to what I am talking about or what I mean. Sometimes she repeats the word 'breakfast' in a monotonous way and gets up.

I tell her to go to the bathroom first and ask, "Maybe you want to brush your hair?"

When she reappears, she has applied lipstick and even her earrings. It all just depends on any given day for the following one might not result in any of the above.

I keep wipes everywhere to sanitize her hands before we have a meal or go out. This point is very important because when she wipes herself in the bathroom, all of her hand and half her arm are 'down there' to get it right. I am blessed for I must admit that I do wonder when the day will come that she cannot take care of herself any longer.

Time to remember to stay in the 'present moment.'

Back to the morning hour with and Joy. Fresh fruit, a toasted croissant, one egg (any style), two or three half strips of bacon are served on the daily breakfast plate.

Yesterday, she ate every bite; this morning I have to feed her all the omelet, plus fruit. Joy stares at the croissant and suddenly scoops it up with her fork, using her fingers to push whatever is left into her mouth. Watching this performance is not a pretty sight, but it works for Joy and her condition.

At the moment, this elegant lady prefers to eat everything on her plate without silverware. Not so with the bread. Taking a roll and applying plenty of cold butter somehow remains her staple in memory.

Joy watches my actions closely to assist her in understanding and executing her task at hand. Even this thinking process seems to be slowly fading. She stares at the TV and forgets the world around her.

Trying to interrupt her forlorn expression, I ask, "Did you enjoy your breakfast?"

Joy slowly lowers her gaze to look at her plate. Sometime it is to eat a bit more, other times there is nothing at all. This can go on for an hour or more. Eventually, the time comes for me to take over and help her finish. Amazingly, she opens her mouth wide like a fledgling while I act as the mother bird.

I tell myself to no longer treat her as a child but as a baby. It is rather challenging to do so for one sees this grown woman sitting there not reacting to anything, just staring blankly at one spot.

When Joy comes from her bedroom and arrives at the table in the kitchen, I have to scoot her close to the table. My hips, back, and arms are definitely being challenged with these motions. Working out and strengthening one's arms and body is a good thing.

It becomes interesting when Joy is ready to leave the table. She has to muster all her force and strength to lift herself up and off the chair. She leans forward, reaches across the table, placing her right hand at the edge, and then pulls.

When I first started caring for Joy, I wanted to do, and did, everything for her. First, out of respect for an elder; second, the fact that she is my employer; third, knowing she has Alzheimer's disease; and last, that it is part of my job. Then I learned from the agencies not to do so for she needs to use every muscle available to her, including her brain. That makes sense to me even though it is difficult to begin with to just stand there and observe. Earlier, she had mentioned to me that I treated her like an invalid.

One evening, after tucking her into bed, she looked at me with a smile and said, "You treat me like a baby."

She is right on. I do what I would do for my

little grandchildren. What is one to do? I decided on a little less tucking.

The challenge for a caregiver is to find the balance between being helpful or letting the patient struggle. Joy is still rather efficient and has the ability to surprise us all.

After breakfast, she routinely takes her meds and goes back to bed. Now I know why the nap. Picking up her meds from the drugstore, I detect a little extra tag on one of the containers: "May cause drowsiness." I have to laugh. This attachment had never previously been on any bottles and not since then, but at least now I know why Joy always goes back to bed and sleeps. Actually, it is the perfect time for all of us. Time for me to clean the kitchen, do the laundry, or just take a break.

About one PM (on my schedule), we have some lunch or a nutritional snack with a glass of milk, including her meds.

No matter what she takes to control the urge of having to go, I still have to find a public restroom every hour to an hour and a half, no matter where we are cruising. After driving for years on the highway south or north, I know a place on every corner where it is convenient for us to stop. Drugstores and fast food places are the most accessible. I am grateful every day to be able to utilize these public facilities. Perhaps my next chapter should be about public restrooms, where to go, and where they are consistently challenging no matter how often I mention this to a manager.

What I do like to mention are the clean restrooms in all the fast food places we have been utilizing on our excursions. In addition to this gratitude list is the fact that Joy prefers restaurant dining and, therefore, we are strictly limited to the toilets everywhere else.

"Time to wash up and get ready," as Joy used to say, "and get out of the house."

Now her pretty underwear has been replaced by pull-up diapers. Sounds simple. A few months ago this was unacceptable; absolutely no way. She was adamant about it. We caregivers had had enough for she could not get to the toilet in time and soiled herself.

It happened on the wooden floor in the kitchen and hallway, along the carpet in her bedroom and all the way into the bathroom, all carpeted in white. Several times I was lucky for the carpet cleaners were scheduled and on their way. Other times I was the one to clean and yet another time I had to call for professional help.

The stench is the worst. I continuously tell myself, "Don't breathe, don't breathe." What I meant, of course, was not to breathe through my nose.

I had thought I would never ever do something like this for anyone but my mother and she passed on before it ever became an issue. There I am — unable to run away and leave Joy to herself, a rather irresponsible and foolish act on my part. Also, I am not a quitter. I recalled all the tasks I had managed during three years as a hotel apprentice in Germany and Switzerland. There is only one thing for me to do. My Alzheimer's patient becomes my mother. From that point on, I have plenty of opportunities to challenge myself with the position.

"Would you have answered your mother like that?" I asked myself this question several times in my mind and always answered by shaking my head.

"Would you have treated your mother like that," I wonder again.

"Yes, I would have, maybe with a little different sound in my voice."

On that note, I recall so vividly my mother's wise remark, "It is the sound that makes the music."

Oh, Mama, you wonderful woman. Mother is always our mother. Please appreciate her while she is alive. We never want to live with regrets that eat one up and eventually make one sick.

"Would you have wanted this for your mother?"

I leave a note for Joy to let her know where I am and when I'll be back for breakfast. With the TV and lights on, she is always content.

When I first started working for Joy, I did ask for permission to leave and go for a run. She actually got a great kick out of this as walking just for pure enjoyment was incomprehensible to her. She laughed every time I returned, especially in winter when my cheeks were cold and red.

Why would one do such a thing?

I had to laugh as well.

Upon my return today, nothing has been touched. I don't like to wake her up for I do believe in the natural course of sleep. She obviously needs the rest. Nevertheless, I feel sad or at a loss for this means that I am slowly losing a friend. Sometimes there is no end to her sleeping and it is time for me to help a bit.

My daughter made some fabulous granola that Joy loves. Now I do the same right here at her home. She also likes store-bought trail mixes, any chips, and salsa with lots of guacamole, and fresh orange slices. We alternate as we go.

Mealtime is every four hours.

Joy eats everything that I eat, which makes life very easy. Sandwiches were not on the menu where I was raised in Germany, so poor Joy just gets them occasionally, the same with French fries. Our lunch consists more of salads, topped with goodies, and I order some chips on the side.

The afternoon is filled with a push in the wheelchair around the beautiful grounds of her neighborhood. Walking was never Joy's favorite for as long as I have known her. After she fractured both ankles (one at a time), she simply does not volunteer to walk more than a half a block and back. Now, during the summer season, we sit together around the pool and she watches me swim and exercise.

"Time to get ready and out of the house," is Joy's favorite expression.

If I now say this to her, I get no reaction or

wink of understanding. Her eyes stare at me blankly.

She showers with guidance and not every day, maybe every second or third day while in my care. Everyone does home care a little differently.

One of my best friend's older husband had Alzheimer's disease. We compared notes many time and concluded that this fetish of daily scrubbing is exactly that — a fetish. How dirty can one get by sitting at home or sleeping? So we wash alternate days at the sink.

Then comes the tooth brushing, which I have to show her by motioning with my arms and mouth to help her remember what to do with the brush. Many times the paste falls off before the ceremony gets under way.

The faucet has to be open for her at all times. I do believe she is so used to having the water running as we did in the days when we gave not the slightest thought as to where the water came from and how precious every drop really should mean to us. The mindset back then was, "If I pay for it, I can do whatever I please with it, right?"

Rinsing and spitting with the water running would go on forever if I didn't finally take the brush away. The residue of the toothpaste, which is now stuck in the sink, gets a continuous rinse with her hand and water, never touching the paste and therefore never getting rid of it.

For me, just standing there watching this scenario day in and day out — over and over again without any changes until I finally interfere and turn off the water — is enough to make anyone jump out of their skin. I sometimes leave Joy and do something else, like brushing my own teeth!

While this is going on, her nose drips almost continuously so I always reach for a tissue and pass it to her. She now does not volunteer her hand but lets me catch the drip.

I am on to her. She just forgets that I expect her outreaching hand to hang on to the tissue. So I point to her hand while shaking my head and smiling. She gets it.

Back to the bedroom and bedside for dressing. It's a ritual by now and I do not want to forget to mention that Joy only has elegant clothing. Undergarments are laid out with her blouse and bra, always a scarf and trousers. We no longer have use for all her belts, matching to every outfit. Having had a very small waistline, Joy looked rather smart with them on.

She is not the only one gaining weight for staying all day in the house lets me constantly open the fridge or cupboards.

Today is the time to stop this snacking and munching. I have had enough. I look at myself and have a good talk with that 'self.' Off to the drugstore. I figured about two weeks of some diet pills will put me on a good track. Almost $30.00 for a bottle. I am getting old(er).What happened to the $5.00 container I used to buy?

"That's ridiculous," my head spills out. "You can do this without all those pills."

So I leave the pills on the shelf and change my eating habits, starting early in the morning. It had become so bad that I stuffed my mouth before leaving the house for a walk. Mostly fruit and yogurt, I have to add.

Time to fix breakfast for the two of us — bacon, eggs, and all the trimmings.

Joy loves chocolate and so do I. 'No mas' in this casa. Cookies and sweets are bought while we stop to go potty, but only for Madame. I mean business. This going out every night for dinner also needs revising. Every other night is plenty and maybe not even that. Preparing our meals from scratch does not make sense any more. Joy does not care at all if our meal is ordered in or prepared by my loving hands. A glass of wine and some conversation have become my imaginary companions. The wine is available; the rest, unfortunately, is not.

Then there are the dirty dishes waiting patiently for my arrival at the sink. Doing dishes or cleaning up after the consumption of a delicious meal has never bothered me. The negative is not having a partner to converse with and appreciate the work that goes into a lovingly and specially prepared meal.

I scrub the pots and pans while Joy instructs me to leave the kitchen as is. All she wants is to be in bed and me lying next to her. Sometimes all this is so small and not worth even mentioning or thinking about; other times, I feel like jumping up and running. Time to laugh at myself and pour a glass of wine.

The question remains: "Running from what, whom, and running to where?" Maybe it is the feeling of quickly running away from myself. Then my savior appears — the reminder! That familiar soft voice:

Change your thinking.
Change your life.

CHAPTER EIGHT

Patience

Life is falling into place.
Keep breathing deeply and meditate.
The rest will flow like the river.

The monotony of caring for an Alzheimer patient day in and day out puts anyone to a test. I say the same things over and over with little or no results. On the other hand, Joy repeats herself constantly and I react, sometimes by raising my voice. When that is over with, I feel badly, apologize, or even cry.

We are together for weeks and months and I don't feel or see any changes until it happens. Whenever we return from an outing, Joy is the last to bolt the door to the garage. One day, she does not. I cannot believe it.

Watching TV later in bed, she asks me if

all the doors are locked and the bolt shut to the garage door as well. From that day on, it becomes hit and miss.

Time to smile, knowing all is well and most of all, time for patience.

Why do we need patience? What is the big deal?

Almost all of my friends, family members, and acquaintances assure me that patience is the one attribute they don't possess.

Why is that? Has progress and our lifestyle changed us so much? Some might reply they never had patience to begin with.

Every time I visit the old country of Germany, I am struck by their driving habits. Those predominantly smaller cars must give the driver the right to slip in and out of spaces like madmen or women. Patience has no chance to appear or develop. The same phenomenon is now happening here in the United States. Smaller and much higher cars than we were used to are everywhere and lead us to the same sporadic actions.

I taught myself patience many years ago. I just did not want to act like a chicken with its head cut off! There were too many of them already. I also had a deep look into myself to analyze what this thing called 'stress' is all about. Everyone seems to use this expression. Many are stressed and become more stressed by affirming over and over how stressed they are.

My answer arrived very clearly. I wanted to become a patient person. By chance, I watched a documentary about Buddhism and two young Buddhists who sat day after day at the roadside, waiting to be admitted for an audition with a sage.

I was fascinated by their patience. This was most remarkable to us Westerners. How can anyone sit by the roadside for days, waiting patiently to be received to accept much longed-for advice?

I also remembered the story of 'young Mohammed' who stood motionless at his father's side day in and day out, waiting to receive his blessings. Unimaginable to relate for his father knew that his son would never return. Those imprints were stuck in my memory bank.

My mind was made up. I would not give anyone, not even the media, the power to influence my life any longer. What a milestone!

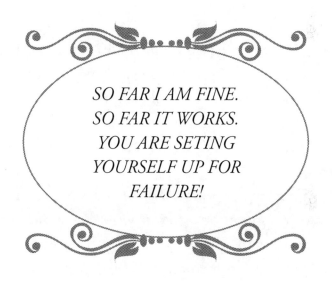

SO FAR I AM FINE.
SO FAR IT WORKS.
YOU ARE SETING
YOURSELF UP FOR
FAILURE!

CHAPTER NINE

Onward

When Joy gets up, which she is still handling on her own, and I hear her approaching with her walker — clunk, clunk, clunk — at times I feel like running away.

"Oh, dear God, how much longer can I do this?"

Then she appears. There is no smile or any kind of motion or emotion visible. The minute I greet her by giving her a hug and a kiss, she reciprocates immediately. When I smile, she smiles back. The poor soul is doing her absolute best with what she is still able to manage. I need a spanking for thinking the way I sometime do.

She does not know how to eat properly any longer. Her fingers are becoming her tools. She makes terrible personal noises. She coughs and spits up right at the dinner table. She clears her throat over and over again. She yawns as loud as she feels like and puts her hand into her mouth to find some dinner residue. If I would see or hear this at a restaurant, guaranteed I would look and smile. No judgment.

It is the daily repetition of those constant, familiar sounds that are so difficult to ignore and that are only asking for understanding. That is all and I still have to pull myself together, not always, by any means, but occasionally. Everything counts and makes me realize how much more there is to do on my part. I compare my growing spurts with a 'seatbelt.' (That device only does us any good if we ALWAYS wear it, not just once in a while.)

Yesterday I walk into Joy's home and observe myself throughout the day.

She comes out of the bedroom smelling of urine. I immediately feel an indwelling resentment. My goodness, I have just arrived. What happened to my resolution? Forgotten are my good intentions, at least for the moment.

Now I am on it. "BE KIND," I say to myself.

I change Joy and remind myself that she 'is' my mother in thought. She acts restless by getting up from her bed, hanging out with me in the kitchen for a few minutes, and then returning to her room and into bed. Back and forth. Back and forth. What is going on in her head?

She falls asleep instantly and wakes up in the same fashion. I check on her and call her name. No answer, no movement, no reply. She is bundled up like a sushi roll in her blanket, just a bit of her white hair visible. Amazingly enough, Joy is breathing regularly and calmly. A minute later she appears, looking at me disparagingly.

She is having a most difficult time formulating what's in her head to make me understand how long she waited for me to enter her bedroom to help her get out of bed. This is my interpretation of her expression on a normal basis. In fact, I know she was just fast asleep a minute ago.

Joy used to tell me daily to wake her as soon as I get up. To miss some activity or anything happening outside her bedroom was almost incomprehensible to her.

Her impatience during the day sets my alarm to keep moving and get ready so we can go for a ride.

I explain to her in charades that I will quickly take a shower. If I speak without using my arms, she will go and sit in her car. If, after a minute or ten, it still feels too long, impatience sets in and Madame might take off, by foot, hopefully. The situation, at this point, is still safe.

Joy resents having to walk — with me or with her walker. Nevertheless, this woman seems to live on resources hidden from all of us. Whenever I make a decision about her condition or restrictions, she gets into action by stepping out for a surprise.

After quickly showering, I come out of the bathroom and there she stands in the middle of my bedroom, clad only in diaper panties with her bra in hand.

"Help me," were the only words out of her mouth.

When her body is washed and the bra fastened, she starts brushing her teeth. This is our daily ritual with the difference that she excludes me today and goes her own way.

"Well!" I think, "I am just going to let her go as far as she is able to handle herself and her attire."

Back in my room, I get ready at top speed. Unbelievably, Joy walks in fully dressed.

I have been dressing her for months, including choosing her outfits, jewelry, shoes, and lipstick.

It was all there. She also walks in without her walker, which is rather dangerous and makes my heart skip a beat.

"Good Lord, help us all!" I pray.

We drive off into another of California's beautiful, sunny days. When we are out together, I always time her 'potty' visits. One hour and a half in between stops is average.

After a half hour of driving, I stop at one of America's favorite stores for some specialty lettuce — an in-and-out situation. I felt safe leaving Joy in the car and quickly run in and out but still not quick enough for her. There she is, crossing the driveway. I have not even paid for our goods.

"You promised to stay in the car," I call out to her.

"I have to go to the bathroom," she replies.

What can one say to that? How long does it take me to realize what's going on in her head? This poor woman is not dealing with the world any longer. She has plenty to do keeping herself afloat.

Her soul is lost. She does not seem to recognize anything any longer. She is confused, which she shares with me. She also tells me that she feels safe with me. Joy is no longer capable of clearly expressing herself, but after she repeats herself over and over again, one gets the idea.

She is happy in my company. Maybe she is saying this to all the others as well. Who knows? She makes it clear to me that all she wants is to go for a ride and look around, not get out, and me being her partner. This feels like going forward. We are growing closer and more intimate. So we forfeit dinner and drive until bedtime.

"I am not hungry," Joy comments after several hours.

I translate this as "keep driving."

At home, the phone rings for me. While talking, I check on Joy and find her curled up and asleep in her bed. Regardless, dinner is on the stove for I am not ready to retire.

Sure enough, a minute later she approaches with a displeased expression, calling out, "I have been waiting for you."

One could easily feel inferior. No doubt, she has her ways. Again, I start laughing but tell her that I had just found her in bed asleep and therefore she could not have been waiting too long.

Am I an idiot?

I did it again.

Joy has no capacity left to understand or comprehend my side of this matter. And what am I doing? I either explain or argue. At least I have learned to do it in a nice and kind fashion.

Oh my goodness, where is my 'embrace'? Where is everything I have learned when something so minute still puts me in a defensive mode? I am ashamed of myself.

Joy sits down and eats. I smile at her. She smiles back. She is happy when I am happy. This is a learning curve for me, another one.

"Move forward," I remind myself.

The decision is made. No more explaining to Joy. No more reacting towards anything coming my way. Only love. That is it.

Love makes the world go round and I know we have so much of it available. Again and again, the same scenario. It is all up to me.

Any moment now, Joy should be coming out of her room and I am happy to see her. How blessed I am to be healthy, wealthy at heart, and wise to realize both. Olé.

Lately Joy fell several times. After fracturing five ribs, she recuperates remarkably well. The danger of pneumonia, however, is imminent. Oxygen is brought into the house. Doctors and therapists make their rounds on a daily basis. Joy likes attention to a point. When this point arrives, she closes her eyes in a way only she can and that everyone understands. Leave me alone.

No need to flip out, have a tantrum, or start screaming. Simply close your eyes and breathe.

All our negative feelings will calm down and come to an end. We have to get better today than we were yesterday. Go forward.

One day Joy and I go out to eat oysters at one of our favorite restaurants. Madame and I are whisked away to our 'usual' table. Fried oysters, topped with the house's special olive relish — it's the best!

After returning home, Joy grows restless. Into bed she goes and then out of bed. Up and down the hallway into my room. Back into her bed and then up again. By now, it is 10:00 PM. No rest for either of us. Off she takes again, this time towards the kitchen. Turning to me, she complains that she is hungry. I don't know if I truly believed my reasoning would alter her determination for it surely did not.

I keep the house dark at night in order to deter her from wandering around. It most certainly did not deter this woman from her mission. She comes back and asks me to show her how to turn on the lights in the living room.

I am stunned. Joy is on a non-stop excursion. She devours the 'tres leche cake' with bananas we brought home as we could not quite finish the huge piece served at dinner. Back to bed she goes.

Not more than five minutes later, the exact scenario.

"I'm hungry. Aren't you?"

I pretend to be sleeping, unsuccessfully, of course, for my Joy is unstoppable.

Time for our second seating in the kitchen, this time with the TV on. It cannot be more than a few minutes before Joy gets up and goes back to bed. Two minutes later, she is standing straight. I hope her aim is the bathroom, but no, she heads towards the bedroom door.

Enough is enough. I run past Joy and close both French doors. While I am expressing my dismay over the evening, or rather the night, I opt to bolt the portal shut. The bolt is all the way at the top of the door and therefore not easy to reach and handle. Joy is much shorter than I am. She would have to stand on her toes to reach that area if, in fact, she is still able to do so.

After we are lying in bed, I finally doze off.

Lucky me, she is up again and trying to get out. In disbelief, I contemplate staying right where I am. Joy is walking, moaning, and groaning. Unfortunately, or fortunately, my Spirit doesn't let me rest. The internal dialog in me has painted a canvas full of mishaps, including her falling backwards, away from her walker. I fly out of my cozy bed and duvet cover to coax her back to bed.

Re-reading these lines, I almost feel a little foolish at writing this episode down, but I do like to share the daily life with an Alzheimer's patient. Joy does get up once more and manages to open the bolt. Unbelievable! I would have bet any amount against this possibility.

After taking a few steps, she turns and exclaims, "I am sick."

So am I.

She is not sucking me into her staying-up-all night mode, or is she? So again, I pretended to snooze off.

"I am really sick," I hear her calling out again.

"Why would she be sick?" I start reasoning with myself.

Then comes a slow and concise sentence out of her mouth. "I don't think you understand my situation."

"You are right, Joy," I respond, feeling rather alert.

I turn towards her, hearing a deep sigh as she calls, "Help me. Help me."

Within seconds I stand at her bedside, looking into panic-stricken eyes.

"I am so sick," is all she can say.

Finally, the oysters pop into my head. That is it! I know that kind of pain. Nevertheless, it has been about seven hours since we ate our early dinner. I run for the chamomile tea and some dry bread for absorption. Nothing helps. A cool towel on her forehead seems to soothe her pain a bit.

I have to admit to feeling rather helpless. She needs to either vomit or sit on the toilet. Unfortunately, she can do neither one. Nothing happens. I suggest and show her how to put her finger in her mouth and throat to initiate some relief. It is too much. Poor soul. She has tired herself out and is now more than ready to fall asleep.

After the intake of some Tylenol, she is finally able to calm down. By 1:00 AM, she is out.

Not trusting her peaceful sleep, I drape towels on the floor and around her, just in case. I cannot understand why she did not feel worse as time went by, the way I remembered my own situation so well.

At last, morning arrives. After assuring myself of Joy's regular breathing and facial color, I sneak out of the room to let her sleep as long as she can.

She comes out of her bedroom at 10:30 AM sharp, looking very fine. She stands in the hallway, grinning, while her face slowly turns ashen.

"I am so sick," is all she can muster, and again that poor woman has to endure the same condition all over again.

While she is trying to sip some Chamomile tea, I brief the arriving caregiver of the night's events. Whatever is in Joy's stomach has to come out somehow, at least that is my way of thinking, but it is not happening.

When I arrive one week later, Joy is still in pain. The doctor was called and more meds prescribed. Her primary doctor advised me to take Joy to the Emergency Room for a CAT scan, just to be sure. There are concerns.

Our regular Urgent Care location does not have a doctor available on this particular day, so I call another clinic. In we go for blood work only, it already being too late to get an imaging appointment.

At 8:00 PM, the doctor calls with the good news that we do not have to go to the Emergency Room after all. Great, for we are lying in our beds, still dressed in case we run out of preferable choices. I have taken Joy twice to the local Emergency Room and vowed not to put her through the trauma of sitting or lying in a bed waiting for hours unless she is in great pain or danger.

Joy seems just fine except when she yells "Ouch!" here and there. The Urgent Care physician mentions 'gall stones' as a possibility and, sure enough, that is what it turns out to be. Surgery, it is decided, is no longer an option. Her diet has to be more bland, fat free, no spices, or nuts.

Joy slowly recuperates, her appetite not the greatest. She has already lost some weight and is now starting to get back into her beautiful wardrobe, which I had sadly stored away in the hall closet. This petite woman begins to look chic again. Her larger-size attire was quite limited with her waistline greatly expanding.

Her butter-less meals are taking care of the rest. White slices of bread slathered with butter were her indulgence. Any chocolate, cheesecake, or ice cream followed the ranks. This can't go on for long.

Remember, caring for an Alzheimer's patient at this stage, there is hardly any recollection. Feeling sorry for this condition only makes the situation heavy and more complicated.

CHAPTER TEN

Oh No, It Happened!

Recently we had a lot of changes. Joy fell and was badly bruised. She was taken to Urgent Care. Nothing broken, thank goodness. A few weeks later, it happened again. This time her fall was much more serious.

When I arrive, she is asleep in her clothes on top of the bed. The other caregiver had her ready to return to Urgent Care where she had been taken the day before after another fall.

Once alone with Joy, I called the doctor for I wondered why we needed to return the day after the incident. The X-rays revealed five fractured ribs, posing a danger zone for contracting pneumonia. We caregivers need to be taught how to do breathing exercises with Joy as her oxygen level has become extremely low.

Just moving her into an upright position at the

edge of the bed is all both of us can handle. She is in enormous pain. I cannot touch her without causing her to scream. The other challenge facing me is my fear that I will make matters worse by moving her through the pain. How in the world has she been handled the previous day getting her up from the fall, into the car to Urgent Care, and then back home and into bed! All I can think is, "That poor woman!"

I call Urgent Care and speak to the attending physician. We decide it is safer to call

9-1-1. An emergency response team arrives in no time and takes good care of Joy. If at all possible, I want to spare Joy a journey to the hospital. I am glad I did what I did. To be honest, there is little that can be done for her. After the diagnosis of her chest X-ray and receiving some short training on how to handle her, we are good to go. The physician explained that she is a 'healing process' patient. The usual procedure is to send such patients to a skilled nursing facility, but in her case, she can return home as long as she has care around the clock. I also receive instructions as to what I can and cannot do. A nurse's aide accompanies us to the bathroom where I learn to work through Joy's occasional pain outbreak and do what has to be done. The assistance and advice are very beneficial.

A social worker initiates all the help available for Joy's in-home care. A commode shows up at the front door. A physical therapist (PT) appears to evaluate Joy and schedule an appointment time. The doorbell rings again, this time a nurse (RN) arrives. Joy's vital signs are taken, evaluated, and noted. Shortly afterward, an occupational nurse (ON) comes to bath and clean her and show us how to be more efficient under the circumstances. Then her primary physician appears for a house call and orders an oxygen machine, just in case. This is enormously helpful.

Madame is Madame and therefore incredible. Within two days, Joy is at it and uses all her might to sit up in bed. This is a major accomplishment for her. She has to be turned from one side to the other. To the right is manageable. Lying on her back seems the easiest and most natural way for her. Towards us is hardly ever successful because she is never far enough into her bed to be turned 180° without the possibility of falling off. Remaining in the same position for too long could accelerate the possibility of her contracting pneumonia for the intake of her breath is much too shallow. We need oxygen!

Practicing deep breathing is, so it seems, a fruitless task. I almost start hyperventilating trying to demonstrate what she has to do. Joy's cooperation is close to zero. We do it anyway. Both of us caregivers made a commitment to do whatever it takes to help Joy out of her danger zone. Anything to battle the chance of getting pneumonia.

When Joy tries to get out of bed, she hangs half way off it towards the floor — not a good thing. The dilemma remains. She has long forgotten her fall and certainly does not know or remember why she is in pain. Any wrong move makes her cry out and sends wondrous looks my way. At night, I jump up when I hear her stir. It happens about every two to three hours, day and night. She is used to making the run to the toilet by herself. She always thanks me for helping her and wonders why I am so attentive. Sometimes I am in a deep slumber and really do not want to get up. Then I hear my little voice (my Spirit) say, "Here is your choice. You either jump out of bed and assist her or you may well end up having to go to the hospital if she falls." Wham! I am out of bed in no time every time.

I am amazed at how exhausting it is when one does not get a good night's sleep. The three-week mark is approaching. I decide to take Joy out for a drive without stopping for dinner. Our undertakings these days are a very slow process. Joy does not remember anything. I motion with my hands to show how to brush her teeth. Joy rinses and spits forever. I finally interfere. I wash her and brush her teeth at the sink and not every day in the shower. All her personal hygiene is now performed by us as well.

To choose her attire and get dressed no longer is of interest to Joy. Sometimes she stands there, looks at herself in the mirror, and actually sees herself. When this happens, she reaches for her lipstick. She tries to keep a straight line but oversteps her contours. Taking her hairbrush, which is always on the vanity, to brush her beautiful white hair, seems to still be a manageable task. I love any action Joy is still able to perform.

When in the car, she always managed to click her seatbelt closed, mostly by the time I am seated. That is now over. For a while, I insisted on her trying harder by letting her fumble and struggle a bit, which she did with success. No more. My inner voice reminds me to be more gentle and understanding. Whatever is most beneficial for her is what counts.

There is total confusion in Joy's head as to which direction to walk. She always knew where we parked her car. Now, she no longer recognizes her automobile and that is big.

Recently, on the way home, we drove around the corner and approached her house. I push the garage door opener, drive into the garage, and turn off the engine. Joy turns to me and speaks quite clearly, "What are we doing here?"

That short remark comes with a deep meaning. I now believe she is no longer able to let us know that she is hungry. She simply would not eat and starve. I am convinced of this.

In the third week after Joy's fall, I take her out for a drive and dinner. She barely eats and takes only a few bites from me as I attempted to feed her, sitting opposite her in our booth. I notice that she has no problem letting me feed her at home. She opens her mouth like a little bird or a baby. In a restaurant, she does not like me to do so. Good. Now I know she still feels the difference. When we arrive home, I serve her some ice cream and a cookie, her favorites. By the time the sun goes down, we are in, or at least on, our beds. Ten PM, lights out, TV off.

My Alzheimer's patient is healing. Joy's pain has lessened and her breathing has improved. She seems so puzzled by all the activity — the hustle and bustle. Though the bones are mending, the mind is not.

It is quiet in the house. During my private time, I turn off the TV and its music. Where is my beloved Beethoven? With his creativity playing in the background, my writing might have a special 'ring' to it.

I finally have to give Joy some stool softener. When does one stop? When an accident happens? It is very apparent that Joy has lost control of this matter. Fortunately, she likes to take a shower. That part is still okay. This way we are able to keep her fresh and clean.

Joy is a member of a local yacht club, which we visit more often now for there are still people who recognize her and the good times they spent together. Someone always comes over to our table to have a little chat with us. Joy can no longer interact but I know she enjoys these social minutes.

Somehow, I believe from the AC in the car, I contract a sore throat. This quickly escalates into misery. I throw myself from one bed onto another. Then, while slumbering, I hear Joy come out of her room, pass me by and dash, with her walker, of course, straight to the garage. Her intent is quite clear to me. She is going to sit in the car.

It's been done before. Fortunately, a good friend of mine whose husband was diagnosed with the same disease told me that he always took off and sat in the car where he waited patiently. You know how active our minds can become, creating a story. Mine is simple. I have her falling down that one step into the garage or losing her footing by having to step up. That is not about to happen. I run to catch up with her. She is already in her seat, staring straight at the blank wall. I open the passenger door and look into that wondrous and wide-eyed face.

Something has prevented the garage door from closing completely. It has closed, just not all the way. Sunlight makes its way in. Joy finally gets out and stops to investigate the calamity. Something is different. She stares at the door, back at me and back at the door again. I start to explain and catch myself just in time. How fruitless such an effort seems anyway.

That night Joy is more restless. She keeps mentioning the garage door and the fact that she has to go close the door and turn off the light. Nothing doing, I reassure her. Every door is securely locked and all the lights are turned off.

Another evening, Joy turns off every light I have just turned on. She tells me, "There is a depression out there."

Another time, while giving her more toilet paper, I received the same warning. "Why do you give me so much paper when there is a depression going on?"

About two AM, Joy gets up. I wait for the sound I am familiar with — pushing the door to the bathroom open. That does not happen. She is off to the garage.

I still keep the house dark at night so she won't be able to see and wander off. The outside lantern must give her enough light to move through the dark kitchen into the connecting hallway, then open the door to the laundry room, pass the ironing board with the iron on top, and move towards the garage door and that critical step down once the door is opened.

I catch up with Joy while she is touching the walls, step-by-step to get to her destination. She becomes frustrated, slapping louder and harder.

"Where is that door," her mind is insisting.

She has miscalculated. Guaranteed that a fall down that deep step would have been imminent. But I reach her in time, observing her actions through the dim light of an electronic device. I plant myself in front of the door and wait for her reaction.

"I need to close that garage door," she keeps repeating.

About two hours later, the whole scenario repeats itself. Back in bed, she actually expresses her thoughts clearly enough for me to understand.

"This is my house. I have to know what is going on in my house. I have to make sure the doors are locked. This is my house. You don't understand what I want."

There you have it. I turn on the light and take a deep breath while grabbing her hand. Then I speak to her.

"Joy, this is why I am here. To keep you safe and secure. If you think you don't need me anymore, I will leave tomorrow. I do not think you want to be in your house all by yourself. Let me know how you feel."

As I speak to her kindly and with love, as I would had she been my own mother, it is interesting how she literally digests our conversation.

She turns and looks at me and holds my hand. "No, don't leave. Stay right here."

About an hour later, she is ready to take off again. I jump out of my deepest sleep as though bitten by a tarantula and block her exit. I have had it. Tougher measures have to be implemented. I lock our bedroom door, which has a huge bolt at the top. Back to bed we go. She cannot rest. After some time, she tries again. (I always have to remind myself that her escapades have already escaped her memory.) There she stands in front of the locked door while I am able to see her silhouette in the dawn light. Eventually, she turns around and goes to bed.

She wakes up earlier than usual, goes to the bathroom and comes out, lipstick on and her top unbuttoned, ready to get dressed and embrace the new day.

She does not mention the garage door again.

The next day, I go out to investigate. The

wastebasket had interfered with the electronics and hindered the door from completely closing. I am glad that chapter is closed.

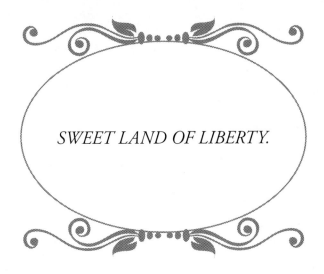

SWEET LAND OF LIBERTY.

CHAPTER ELEVEN

A New Day

Every time I return to take care of Joy, it feels like coming home again. This time, of course, I refer to Joy's house as my second home. The minute I enter through the doorway, I realize a 'newness' all around me. Everything feels different — unfamiliar. Change is in the air; something I cannot grasp or connect to, a coming and going like the changing of the tide. There is a sense of stillness, too still for me to feel comfortable. My guard is on high alert while I tiptoe along the tiled wooden floor.

The flow of energy and vibration in this home has become stagnate. I know the house and feel it. It is communicating discomfort and alerting me from every direction of this solidly built structure. I feel an immediate urge to do something, an inside upwelling to act, to contribute with my 'good stuff' by defusing as much as possible without having to feel sapped afterward.

Joy is different as well. It is the way she approaches me, her look, which turns into a gaze. A stare instead of an acknowledgement upon my arrival is all I receive. Usually, I am greeted with her bright and glorious smile. Emptiness is all I find. I don't think she recognizes me at all and just goes through motions without thought or purpose. Lost. Her answers, whenever she is able to do so, are programmed and consist of a time gone by. That is the difference. A shift in her level of awareness.

Joy and I have the same activities and routines during the week. The realization that it is purely up to me as to how colorful our days can be is wearing me out. Joy will come along wherever I intend to go with her. That she assures me of over and over again. So why am I creating such a big deal? Change is up to me, again.

It is really sweet for her to say this. We do have a good time together, regardless of our old routines. Well, hold on. Not quite.

That's the challenge. She still tells me to go anywhere I choose to drive, to take care of whatever I need to as long as she does not have to participate. She insists on staying in the car while I do the errands. There is a stubbornness hiding deep down in her being that is working its way up to the surface. "I don't want to," is the message. Only when I look at her do I see the Joy of now, the Alzheimer's patient who is not sure of herself at all and just reacted to a command, released by her memory. Being in the enclosure of her car gives her a sense of security. She could sit in there and go for a ride from morning to night, without much food and just an occasional stop for the toilet.

At times, when I know what I need to shop for and can manage it fast, fifteen minutes at the most, I do just that. Any longer will test her sense of loneliness and patience. Oh well, she does not have any of the latter, so let's call it 'impatience.' Joy has never had any patience, at least not during the time I have known her.

With a closer look at my family and friends, I conclude that neither do they. Nothing new here for almost exclusively everyone I share my work experience with reveals their 'impatience' and also 'wish' they had more of it. How crazy is that? Like I was born with an extra ton of it? Patience, like many other attributes is a conscious choice. We bring with us onto this planet earth the seeds of our desires. Pretty fantastic!

I mentioned patience in taking care of an Alzheimer's patient and a new day. When I feel a bit down about myself and the situation at hand, I toil with the overwhelming feeling of not wanting to handle this task. Then, in an instant, I make the decision to be the best I can be. Just going through the motions, resenting what I have to do, or simply sticking to the thought of not liking the work I have chosen to perform becomes unacceptable.

With an Alzheimer's patient, one must stay alert at all times. I did not find this too difficult for I had plenty of time to move into the situation. I assume the same from you in dealing with a family member. The job becomes more demanding as time goes by and conditions change, mostly in an unfavorable direction.

It is now obvious that Joy's awareness has shifted more inwardly. This is the time for more love; the time for more joy, understanding, compassion, and care to get her into a mode of her own acceptance.

We can all do it. We are all made of the 'stuff' to handle what lies ahead. The key is to challenge oneself and not the situation at hand. No doubt, running a household with an Alzheimer's patient as a family member is an enormous daily task and you might hear from your family and friends about 'how' strong you are. You also are made a 'special person' for having all that patience.

"I could never do what you are doing," comes out of almost everyone's mouth as the oldest, simplest, and compassionate statement. To put this 'job' aside for people who are just born with all those positive attributes, a caregiver exerts attributes we all possess.

This scenario is all-inclusive for, without a doubt, my thoughts used to be on the same page: I could never do that kind of a job. Now, I feel blessed all over again to have started this journal and have the opportunity to be able to put some time aside to express my life experiences and help humanity at the same time. That is worth living for. The rest will fall into place.

My mother always used this quotation:

"The magic lies in the details,
The end result will take care of itself."

There are seven TV monitors in Joy's home. Three are in constant use every day and into the night. It is a matter of hearing the noise and watching the action that Joy has to have as part of her wellbeing. Therefore, we all live under the unwritten house rule.

Some time ago, while Joy slept, I started listening to the music channel. When she appeared to join me for a chat or meal, I switched to something I felt was more interesting to her. That does not matter anymore. It is all gone. She is not able to follow a story, the news, or a movie. She asks often for an explanation, mostly when commercials are screeching at a higher volume. I quickly realize her true purpose. She needs my attention and the sound of my voice, not really my thoughts.

Conversation at this stage is the most important matter in her life.

"Talk to me."

"Don't ignore me."

"I am important."

"I have to be important to someone, anyone, to anybody, please."

THOSE ARE HER TRUE FEELINGS.

Family and friends, make sure you visit. The more, the merrier.

Joy can no longer express her pleasure and delight in anyone's presence. It is the only thing she cares about — family, friends, and people who acknowledge her. And, of course, going for a ride in her car.

No one else is with Joy on a daily basis except another caregiver and myself.

The telephone was once her lifeline. She was drawn to it like a magnet. Upon returning home from our nightly excursions, her first glance was to the phone and the answering machine with its blinking light. Had someone called her? That, unfortunately, is passé as well. She likes to listen to the caller but cannot respond, which seems to extremely frustrate her. She gives the receiver back to me or just hangs up herself.

Family visits and get-togethers are more directed towards holidays and birthday celebrations.

Joy is now ninety years of age. She has a bad stumble the day before Christmas. A week after the holidays, she falls again (this time on my watch).

Two weeks into her recuperation from her

previous accident, it happens again. This time she loses her balance while maneuvering her walker up a staircase. My huge mistake was that I ran ahead of Joy to put down some bags before attending to her needs. I hear a 'thump' and literally flew to her side, only to see her lying on her back with her head stretched forward and her arms entwined in her walker.

With enormous cooperation on her part, Joy and I crawl onto a chair where I suggest she sit down and catch her breath. Nothing doing. She pressed on to make it up that fateful step and did not stop until she was on her bed. Something in me feels thrilled for she has just proven that nothing is broken. Again, my concern is directed towards the hospital. Shall I or shall I not call the paramedics or take her to the ER? Clearly, I have to treat her as I would my beloved mother. I decide to observe her for the evening and pay close attention to her condition.

While Joy sits on the toilet, I automatically begin to rub her back, which must make her feel very good. She cannot get enough of it so, well into the night, I continue rubbing when she returns to her bed until she falls asleep. Incredible! No side effects. This certainly teaches me a lesson.

Always, without exception, just like the seatbelt in our cars, we caregivers have to stand behind our patients in order to be instrumental in an emergency.

When Joy starts moving, she advances without being deterred. She can hear us calling her but does not understand. All our screaming to make her come to a STOP is fruitless. A two-year-old displays the same frame of mind. We have to remind ourselves to treat the daily interactions with Joy in retrospect.

Then she falls again! I can imagine the caretaker in charge watching in horror as she lifts up her walker, loses her balance, and falls backwards onto the concrete. The result? A bloody head and a rather upset lady. A call is made to 9-1-1. Into the hospital again. All necessary tests and X-rays are performed. The patient miraculously survives without much harm. Ice packs are prescribed on a constant basis. More ice for the area around her right eye, which is swollen like a water balloon.

Tylenol, if necessary, for her pain or as a calming agent is added to her three medications that she takes on a regular basis. The woman is amazing!

Can you believe that our dear Joy became indignant at the hospital?

"Why are we here? Let's get out of here."

Back in her car, on the way home, she complains of hunger.

"Let's go to dinner. I am starving."

Is that not remarkable? No pain for this lady. She has no recollection of her fall. Over and done.

Needless to say, she is taken home and is well cared for.

When I arrive, I look at the exterior of our patient and find her quite all right. Nevertheless, as the day progresses and her eye starts to swell in record speed, I realize the severity of her condition. Her poor body must still be in shock. So we stay home and hang out together.

Joy shows no special interest in my culinary extravaganzas and, come to think of it, rightly so. Who needs to concentrate on a delicious piece of meat when the body and head are aching? What a shock she has sustained. Time to stay home for more T.L.C.

This cannot happen again. Imagine how awful it feels when the patient so suddenly loses her balance and one is not there to prevent a fall. That is a major part of a caretaker's responsibility — to keep her safe and out of harm's way. Time for a good long look at my inner 'self.'

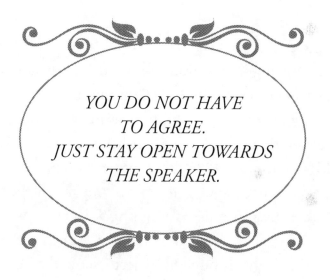

YOU DO NOT HAVE
TO AGREE.
JUST STAY OPEN TOWARDS
THE SPEAKER.

Chapter Twelve

We Are Losing

Yesterday, I walk into Joy's house, see her sitting in her usual spot in the kitchen, and experience a sinking feeling in my stomach. She sits slouched over, looking up at me without any recognition. I walk over, give her a big hug and a kiss on the cheek, longing for her famous smile. She does not respond until I stick my face literally into hers, grinning as brightly as I can muster. It works, but only for a moment. Staring at or staring right through an object is now the norm for her.

After sitting for a while, she tries to get off her chair, a motion she performs in vain and a signal to help her out of her confinement. I have just taken the area rug to the garage as Joy keeps getting stuck on the edges. It is so testy to have to watch her as she painstakingly, in slow motion, does whatever she decides to undertake. We all realize that, throughout our lives, the little things we are pushed to encounter are the most challenging moments to combat.

During a car ride, I ask Joy to pass me a tissue. The box has been forever on her side on the floor. Now, the box has been kicked around and I am unable to reach past her legs. It is not safe to do so and I ask Joy. Watching her go through the effort inch-by-inch, millimeter-by-millimeter, reaching forward and down towards the little shred of white lurking out of the box makes me want to scream. I finally to pull over, loosen her seatbelt and let her complete this arduous task as giving up is not in the cards. She does it!

You may wonder why I don't just take care of this and forget all the struggles. It would simplify matters. Yes, that is the easy way and I used to do it all. I have been advised by the medical profession not to be so active in the care of an Alzheimer's patient. I need to stand back as much as possible in order for Joy to keep her muscles flexible and moving. In earlier years, this was particularly challenging for I saw her as an elderly woman while I am twenty years younger.

I look at Joy as though she is my mother — with

love and respect, wanting to do everything for her. In fact, she told me more than once that I treat her like an invalid. She meant it in a nice way for she smiled as she spoke. I have never forgotten this. Yes, of course, I want to open the door for her. Certainly I run to open the gate to the house. Naturally I reach out to help whenever I have a chance. That is what we do as people in general. We help each other.

When Joy arrives for a meal at the dining area next to the kitchen, we have to scoot her in close to the table. It is quite difficult for her to push herself away and get up without any assistance for her strength, plus her stubborn insistence, is subsiding. By trying to lift herself out of the chair and stand up, back into the chair and up again, we know Joy is ready to leave the table. She is unable to complete this task any longer. Together, we accomplish her desire to return to her comfort zone — the bed.

Off we go and I stay with Joy to guide her back into her bedroom. When I do, we move a little faster. I place myself in front of her walker and pull. I always have to grin while moving along. Joy walks so slowly by herself that it looks absolutely comical when her legs now have to lay on a bit more tempo.

When walking by herself, she looks at every angle of her home, taking it all in and giving me a most forlorn glance. "Where am I? What is this that you call my home?"

Joy is back in bed. No formulated expressions. No sound until I hear an awful yawn. Not a normal yawn. No, a terrible yowling. Standing at her side and listening, I realize that she has added new sounds. In bed, while walking or sitting on the toilet, in the kitchen or the car, she constantly exudes terrible noises. No more mumbling. No effort to compose a sentence or formulate a thought. Just noises.

We have an early dinner and go for a long walk through the neighborhood with Joy in her wheelchair. I have this style of an outing down pat for Madame has her way of complaining.

We are on our way. I am prepared with her cashmere sweater and a blanket on my arm, knowing her overture, "It's freezing out here."

A ray of sunshine, on the other hand, while we are on foot, is enough for her to want to turn around or give a suggestion for a ride in the car. Not yet. We now have visors for the two of us.

It sounds like I have just discovered this handy accessory. Not quite. We used to have a plethora of them in the house as Joy was an avid golfer. In recent years, she refused to wear one so I eventually gave them away to the Goodwill.

The outside temperature has to be comfortable. Going out in the rain is a privilege I bestow on myself. Maybe one has to come from a different climate zone for Southern California does not grow too many 'rain lovers' unless their lawn receives a free watering. Water or rain is, and has always been, so precious to me. I have never understood this kind of negligent behavior or attitude of disliking rainy days or finding the wet climate an inconvenience. When the rain arrives and I talk to the folks on the street, they all chime in with the general 'need' of those drops but unanimously agree, "on second thought, I don't like the rain," final answer.

After one particular outing, we enjoy my Alzheimer patient's favorite ice cream and prepare to retire. Finally, we are both tucked away in bed but there goes my Joy getting out of her bed while I observe her movements. Her aim is not in the direction of her bathroom. She walks straight to the window opposite the foot of her bed, parks the walker, and pushes herself away. She squeezes between a chair and the window, loosens the blinds, and lets them swoop down. Stepping back, and totally freestanding, she starts to walk over to my side of the bed and that window, ready to execute the same maneuver.

Joy looks at her walker as her 'life line and savior.' She won't look up or make one step without this balance bar. She is having a 'moment' of intent, an act of mind, which freed her of her limitation. That is fascinating for me to see and realize.

What do I do? I jump out of my bed and block her way. Wow! Out comes the old Joy. She lifts her arm, ready to hit me or maybe just to warn me off. I grab her wrist, which is not difficult at all. I look into her face and eyes while she expresses sheer anger, topped with ugly yelling. I remember to smile and speak calmly.

She starts to relax, turns around, and goes back to bed without losing the grip of her look at me. Slowly and gently I speak to her, explaining why I want the blinds up for we need airflow throughout the heat wave. I shake my head for I am aware of the fact that Joy does not understand or comprehend my reasoning. Above all, I am not to try to reason with her anyway.

Joy no longer leaves her bed unless we come and get her. She would stay in her bed day in and day out. She would stop eating and starve.

She still uses the toilet but less and less. She forgets why she is sitting on the commode and therefore gets up and leaves. The previous night, I realized from the moment she disappeared to the toilet and returned to bed took no time at all. What is happening? She does not pull her underwear down, sits for a short moment, if that, and comes right back to bed. Her short-term memory is getting shorter.

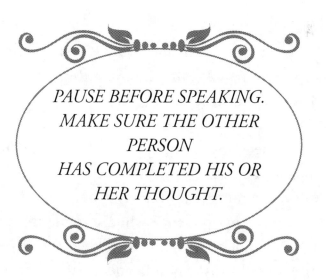

*PAUSE BEFORE SPEAKING.
MAKE SURE THE OTHER
PERSON
HAS COMPLETED HIS OR
HER THOUGHT.*

CHAPTER THIRTEEN

Advancement

Dear Joy is advancing into a baby stage. More and more I realize how little I know about Alzheimer's disease.

One moment she leaves her conscious world and the next minute she expresses herself in a full sentence. She is in bed next to me when she asks, "Are you coming . . .? [into my room]. Somehow, she realizes my presence while formulating the question and lets it fizzle out. Then she covers herself up, turns around, and pretends to go to sleep. I truly believe she felt some sort of embarrassment. After a few minutes, she appears and all is well and forgotten.

Going to the toilet is still part of her exercise but wiping herself is another story. We have taken over brushing her teeth for she gives more attention to wetting the toothbrush and unloading the paste. It is rather amazing how cooperative she is by opening her mouth to let us successfully aim at every nook and cranny we are pleased to attack.

By the time I arrive one morning, Joy has already returned to her bed. I walk into the bedroom, deciding to make it a grand entrance if only for the energy it will create. With much noise and fanfare, I dance into the room, a rose in my mouth and arms flinging through the air. Joy loves it and returns the favor with a big, happy smile. Action and participation seems to always work wonders. It interrupts the monotony. Hours later, she comes up with some comment of approval. We look at each other and smile. All is well.

The staleness in Joy's home can easily get the better of me. It is up to us caregivers to come up with a positive change. Noise is good. Favorable noises like laughter and music are even better. The music selections on TV, especially the symphony channels, are, in my opinion, much to be desired. I love classical, light classical, symphonies, piano concertos, Latin, salsa, jazz, rock and roll, in short, all kinds of music with the exception of heavy metal. Whatever is available creates pain in my ears. No matter how often I listen and switch the channels — and there are many — most of the time I end up turning the whole thing off.

Autumn is in the air at last. A bit cooler, fresher, and most colorful everywhere I turn. We prepare for Thanksgiving and Joy's birthday party.

She prefers to stay in bed all day long and always looks wondrous when I help her get up for a change of scenery. She goes to the bathroom only whenever she has a moment or recollection.

Time for something to eat. As always, I walk behind her to the table and let her slide into her seat. She is very good at that and handles this repetitious task very well. One morning I walk past Joy towards the laundry room and upon my return find her nearly ready to slide down from the chair onto the floor. Only one side of her butt is seated and one leg dangles over the armrest. Even this simple task of sitting down on her chair now needs supervision.

Breathing has become more difficult for she somehow attracted an infection and has been put on several antibiotics. Her blood work is okay so why does she have pain in her side here and there? Gall stones. Strict low-fat diet, no nuts, and plenty of chocolate (just kidding) is the rule. Joy loves chocolate in any form and flavor. I make it my business to keep a good supply at hand. Her face brightens up at the sight. Time for me to unwrap the sweets for Joy tried to put the whole package in her mouth. On that note, the patient is doing well and moving along without all that chocolate.

A new and more high tech walker with a 'ready seat' arrives one day. I cannot possibly see Joy being able to handle this 'fast forward' apparatus. It moves much too easily and therefore will run off with or without her. Maybe I am too cautious? Maybe not. The walker is parked in the garage.

When we are out and about, Joy no longer asks me to make stops for the toilet. What a relief. I cannot even tell you what it means to transport her to various restrooms. We caregivers had our special places, depending on the direction of the daily excursions. Frankly, I could write a book about the condition of those restrooms, combined with the cooperation and excuses of diverse companies. The location of said facilities seems to be a vital factor in cleanliness; some were quite bad! We have overcome that hurdle.

Most recently, Joy sleeps through the night. Fantastic! One night she wakes up, gets up by herself (one of my eyes opened), and goes into her bathroom, only to come back in almost an instant. What was that" She did not even go. The next morning I watch the same scenario. Head towards the toilet, turn around with her walker, sit down, maybe, get up, and back to bed. Apparently she does not remember what to do when she arrives at her destination. That is something we can all relate to.

For a second time I am awakened at night by Joy's feet. She works herself into a horizontal position in bed with her head almost hanging off to the side and her feet digging into my hip. This yanked me out of my slumber. I have to admit that it is a strange feeling when someone else's feet and wiggly toes poke an unprepared sleeper. A hospital bed might have to be the next move. We shall see.

Just dream yourself into the infinite, Joy. The kind of person she projected throughout her life, combined with her stubbornness, I am sure are the key ingredients to her still hanging on. I can't help feeling this way and so wish for her to be able to let go and move on to another plateau. I mentioned my feelings about this subject to another caregiver who was horrified.

Joy has quite a Thanksgiving week, spending it with her family, followed by the excitement and preparation for her ninetieth birthday. Joy is twenty years my senior and a fierce reminder to me to keep moving. (Taking a walk rather than a nap and it works.) Keeping my mind active and in tune, in spite of traces to the contrary, is another challenge I decide to take on. One needs to stay informed by tuning in, not tuning out. I meet so many elderly people who just don't care any more. With this in mind, stagnation arrives. Envision a drifting boat and you know it will eventually sink. We don't have to go overboard or get fanatic. No, just keep one's eyes and ears open and stay on a mission of discovery.

I took some time off from caring for Joy and am shocked upon my return. She did recognize me, smiling briefly. It always takes a day to get her used to the routines involved. This time I find myself shaking my head constantly in disbelief. What has happened? She seems to have forgotten everything there is to know about life.

There is no recognition of her hairbrush, earrings, favorite lipstick, clothes, fork or spoon. No use of her hands in any way but reaching for her walker. I resign myself by realizing the time has come to completely take over her daily way of life. I move over next to her chair to enable my feeding her more easily. Joy is a good eater, especially when a variety is being served. I make up my mind not to have her lose weight on my watch. She sits, sighs and yawns most of the time and closes her eyes between bites.

Giving her a shower is still okay. She has become more insecure and fixes her eyes on mine. Her movements are extremely slow. It feels like she is contemplating every single step.

The two of us used to play solitaire. It was interesting to observe how she tried so hard to put it together. A few weeks ago she still had it. This is also over. Our communication is now shifting from vocal sounds to eye contact. The best deed I am able to give her is a smile. She returns it right away while looking deeply into my eyes.

At breakfast one morning I caressed her hair and told her that all is in order. We looked, blinked, and smiled. I think of the thousands of people in her condition who are dependent on institutions and their employees. Caring for an Alzheimer's patient certainly tests a caregiver's patience, or better yet, teaches patience. Joy is a very sweet soul and ever so helpless. What a blessing for her to receive all our love.

The more love we give, the better the atmosphere in the house. The infinite pool of love is inexhaustible and available to all. I give and take for I don't want to miss out on life. Faith, trust, hope, joy, kindness, and compassion all translate into Love. Let's feel enriched by splurging and giving all that love away.

CHAPTER FOURTEEN

Here We Are

One morning I arrived to a big disappointment. Absolutely no recognition from Joy.

She lies in bed, napping or rather, dozing away. My appearance includes a grand entrance (ta dah!), which usually evokes some kind of a reaction. No matter what kind of face I produce for her, it does not work.

The day goes on as usual. I get Joy out of her comfort zone, the bed, and bring her out to lunch. More and more she eats just a little and then tries to leave her chair and me to go back to bed. I truly believe it is one of the few actions she still remembers. Other than that, she loses interest or forgets why she is here and stares either at her food, the TV or out the window.

I, on the other hand, need to be validated for my creativity in preparing our lunch. It is just a little selfishness coming through. Obviously, I enjoy what I am doing and I do love to cook. Having a customer or guest who does not join in with my passion is a letdown. I end up eating twice as much as is good for me and, on top of it, I have to clean up and do the pots and pans. Will I ever learn?

I make a decision to feed Joy from now on for nothing is wasted on my watch. Sounds rather controlling or, as my husband would say, "So very German." He is probably right!

When Joy sees a sandwich, she goes for the attack. *What about the greens*? I ponder. Here is my chance. I load up her fork with salad greens and she opens her mouth wide like a big bird, inviting every bit without discrimination. The minute I leave her to herself, she acts out on whatever is still in her consciousness. Pushing her plate away, an action I personally dislike, is a clear communication.

"This is it. I have finished." I get it but this isn't it for me.

Now my childhood appears loud and clear or is it my ego?

"Every bite on the plate has to be eaten before one gets dessert or leaves the table." Those words coming out of my mouth have to sound foreign to Joy.

"No, no, Joy. You are going to finish your meal," I hear myself calling out in a nice way and with a smile.

I can still hear my beloved grandfather expressing those words, probably taught to him when he was a little boy. Good traits or bad traits, without evaluating our thoughts and actions, we just go on and repeat.

The look I receive from Joy is priceless. Actually, it is a wondrous expression, like, "I don't recognize this command," and for an add on, "I don't believe I am hearing right."

So I placated myself in front of the mirror, mimicking the way I projected my idea to Joy. There is nothing else I can do but laugh for I do look scary and rather frightening, hovering over her like a towering inferno. At my present stage of life, mindfulness has to be incorporated like taking a breath of fresh air, always and without stopping.

I feed Joy as fast as she can chew for when her mind wanders off, the end is infinity. Tricking her into eating only has a momentary effect. We spend our days in a rather mundane fashion. Realizing that Joy understands more than meets the eye shows up when we are out to dine. I may cut up her meat or break up her roll to butter it, but that is about it. She does not like to be fed or receive any kind of assistance. She waits for me to start eating so she can copy my movements. There, again, this might not represent the norm for we have experienced by now that whenever I think I have figured her out, I am at the losing end.

On a recent day, we went for lunch at a Japanese restaurant where we were served the salad and soup at the same time. Joy did not spare a moment looking at me but took the little bowl with the greens and dumped it into her miso soup. Bon appetite! She ate it all. My grandchild Camille was with us. We caught each other's eyes and giggled.

It is just a learning curve to realize again how minimal and non-important those little ways about us are. So the salad went into the soup. Envisioning a mother in a restaurant with her children, I almost see the horror in her face if one of her children acted likewise, not realizing this banality. We mothers are constantly on our children as far as behavior is concerned. Once in a while, we are at liberty to 'let it go' and smile. Contemplate your reactions towards your husband and children. It's worth the extra minute and effort. This could happen to anyone and most of us mothers would have a fit watching our little ones (unless they were very little) pour soup into their salad or vice versa.

Early in the mornings, I take my walk around the island. A multitude of people are walking, running, phoning, jogging, talking, drinking coffee, and coming out of their homes with their pets in tow. It's active and glorious.

We have, or better, I have, shied away from visiting the Island at dinnertime for the parking availability is rather limited. Yesterday I find a perfect spot. Joy gets to sit in her wheelchair and I have the privilege of getting my exercise. The air is balmy, a little bit like Hawaii, just not as humid. Wonderful. So we take the trip around the island, which is quite a hike. I made sure Joy went to the toilet before we departed.

Would you believe that at the onset of this trek she comes up with her familiar phrase, "I have to go to the bathroom."

Here I am, absolutely loving the present moment and this special time of the evening and Madame has nothing to tell me but that! We finally arrive at the little market on the peninsula site — no bathroom. Onward. My mind unsuccessfully keeps bombarding me not to care. I tell myself that she is wearing a diaper and whatever happens will happen. The concern I harbor is more the Number Two possibility. Now I am pushing faster and faster, telling Joy we are almost there.

"Where is it? When is it coming?" her voice drifts faintly to my ears.

Oh gosh, such a special hour. "Detach. Detach," I say aloud. "Enjoy as much as you can!"

It has to be Spirit reminding my Soul to breathe and enjoy, breathe and enjoy. Olé! It works.

People sit on the beach with a picnic; on the sea wall with an appetizer and a glass of wine; cook delicacies in their open kitchens; or eat dinner on their patios.

Every island houses an artist/painter and there he is. My glance toward his creations interprets more toward an advanced beginner. Is there such an expression?

Children are everywhere enjoying family, beach, and their toys, not to forget the temptation of ice creams and frozen bananas lurking at every corner.

Once we take care of the 'emergency,' which isn't one, we mingle with the immediate world, stop, indulge, and hang out until the sun is ready to say 'good night.'

Being pushed in the wheelchair, not knowing what and who passes her by along the boardwalk simply does not agree with Joy. She also has no idea how long our excursion will last, which gives her a feeling of losing control.

When she does not like a situation, she always has a way of interfering. She never likes walking, requiring that I drive around parking lots in the hunt for a closer place to park. She never wants to sit outside for fear of a bug or a breeze messing up her perfectly coiffured hair. Rolling down a window of her car (even a half an inch) while driving is against the law. Not a minute sound escapes her sharp ears. Her mind seems to be more active than mine for whatever she puts together works. This time she successfully employs the bathroom technique.

Another little anecdote to share. My oldest daughter arrives to take care of Joy for twenty-four hours. She helped a few years ago when Joy was still in good shape. There is a lot going on in this house and a lot to tell. Somehow, I decide to shortcut the training by suggesting that she treat Joy as she would her own grandmother. My daughter is the best person to have around when one is not feeling good and needs care. She is compassionate and an excellent cook. She also seems to intuitively know what someone needs, when someone needs it, and then delivers. So I knew Joy was in the best of care.

My daughter reports, "Joy sure smiles a lot."

When the time comes for personal hygiene, Joy takes the washcloth out of daughter's hand and cleans herself, again with a smile.

Since Joy's tooth brushing is not that good any longer, we caregivers have to do the brushing. She opens her mouth willingly to let it happen. Not this time. Joy takes the toothbrush out of my daughter's hand and performs rather well. Is she fooling all of us?

We decide Joy needs a haircut. To start out, she must shower and shampoo her hair. I do not go into the stall with her for she can still function and wash herself most of the time. The other caretaker always puts on her bathing suit to give Joy a good scrub. My daughter is ready but Joy is not. She does not want a shower, does not need a shower, does not care about her hair, and refuses to cooperate with our plan.

I receive an SOS call from my daughter, who is standing there in her bathing suit without a customer.

My advice? "You have a toddler at hand. Be the mom and know what is the right thing to do for your child. Joy wants to win and I am sure she has done so all her adult life."

After much tricking and determination, mission accomplished!

The same scenario happens with her meals. I am back and end up feeding Joy most of her breakfast. Is it I who cannot stand having her just sit and moan and yawn on a nearly constant basis?

She eats for my daughter. Not as much and for sure on her own time, but she does eat.

The previous night we go to dinner at our favorite restaurant in town. Our server split one of their wonderful salads for the two of us, perfectly presented in a bowl. I add a roll with a little butter on it and watch Joy perform. She lifts her hand with her fork and eats just like everyone else. Amazing.

Joy must be going 'in and out' of herself. Awake, in a slumber, or absent? May she be blessed.

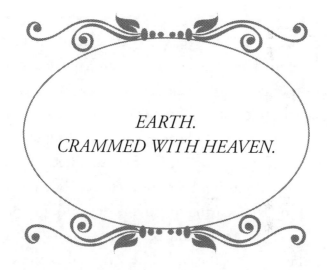

EARTH.
CRAMMED WITH HEAVEN.

CHAPTER FIFTEEN

Good Night My Dear Friend

The past few weeks can be compared to a constant rollercoaster ride. Knowledge is very useful and rewarding. Awareness just arrives as a reminder of my prediction — my dear Joy leaving this form of life on earth. Who am I to say? This has been going on for the last three to four months and during every new episode of change, I feel Joy is preparing to close her eyes for good. I keep comparing her way of being with that of my Mother towards the end of her physical existence.

I leave the house and say good bye to my now dear friend, wondering if I will ever see her alive again. Four days later, I return and there she is, greeting me with a radiant smile of delight to be able to go for a ride. I end up just standing there in disbelief, shaking my head, and adapting to the newly won situation until next time.

Next time is here. Joy has been falling frequently, which is sad and painful for us helpers as well. Amazingly enough, her bones seem to be made of steel and if I didn't know better, deem them unbreakable.

One day last week, Joy's restlessness overcomes her and remains all day and throughout the night. The constant trying to get up to go to the bathroom, living room, into the kitchen (she claims she is starving even though she ate dinner), or just following her inner urge to move, makes the night an unfriendly mate.

When Joy is in bed, she likes to curl up and dig her legs into her covers without stopping until I get to feel her feet in my bed. Out of bed I jump to straighten her legs and tuck in the sheet, blanket, and duvet cover as tightly as possible between our two twin mattresses. For some reason, I have to perform this task several times during the night, including feeding her again and giving her liquids to drink. Then I start, for my sake, meditating like a mad monk with my mantra of ohhhm, ohhhm, ohhhm.

Going back to sleep seems a dream or two away. Slumbering for a few minutes is all I can attain for Joy is on her way up again. Letting her do what she feels she has to do is risky for she constantly loses her balance, trips over her own two feet and stumbles, even with her walker. Finally, the morning hour twinkles through the blinds to announce the arriving day. Joy goes out like a light.

She, in her condition, has no recollection of her falls and wonders about her black, blue, and yellow eye, plus the many bandages on both arms. When the nights are too long and not interesting enough for Joy, she takes the time to peel off her facial band-aids, millimeter by millimeter, while lying in bed. Then she proceeds with her arms and legs.

I get on the phone and order a railing to be attached to Joy's bed. This so desirable item, for reasons not known to us, does not arrive and we change our minds and consider a hospital bed.

It is quite astounding that Joy still has such a good appetite. I do baby her while I am with her for the three days, feeling that this is the right way to go about her wellbeing. She is simply not able to stand on her own feet for more than a few seconds, which makes me literally push her onto the bed to avoid collapsing with her right on the spot. What an undertaking. I decide to learn fast and go through this only once.

Joy is hungry so off to the kitchen I go. Just as I complete my creation, I spot her at the corner of the hallway. Believe me, a ghost could not cause me a more stunned expression. This could not be. I just experienced her not being able to walk another step. I thought her condition to be more or less permanent.

I drop the kitchen tools and run, give her a big smile and guide her towards the table and her chair. There she sits for about a minute or two. One bite is all she can muster. She keeps rubbing her eyes and forehead and expresses a feeling of nausea. Oh, 'lieber Himmel,' this does not sound good. We walk back to her bed and I give her two Tylenol, which helps her into a short snooze. While I contemplate the options available for my next step, she opens her eyes and smiles.

"I feel much better now,"

No dizziness and no desire to sleep. What a relief it is. My only concern is to be able to spare her a visit to the ER. In an emergency, of course, this is where I will take her. How fortunate we are to have nurses and physicians available and ready to assist in her wellbeing. The crisis is past. Time to move on.

Joy stays awake all of this particular day and all night as well — a never-ending restlessness and the desire to get out of bed. Three times, she digs into my bed, her feet pushing into my hip. Between five and six o'clock, I finally pass out and awake close to nine. I turn immediately to look into Joy's staring eyes. She closes them and keeps on slumbering until I wake her for breakfast.

Something needs to be done. On my next visit, we definitely decide on a hospital bed. Unfortunately, Medicare does not cover this expense no matter how great our desire. First, we have to have an accident, then the proper help.

In our case, Joy constantly tries to get out of bed, stumbles, and falls. I suppose that is permissible. Frankly, I don't want to get into this any deeper than I already am. I discuss the dilemma with her physician, who concludes to opt for sleeping pills. The pharmacy, only about three minutes from the house, is open until ten PM. Plenty of time.

Joy does not eat lunch or dinner. She enjoys a ride in her car and gives it all she's got by trying to read the neon signs. She is amazed at the lighted world around her and seems just as surprised to have to get out of the car once I park in the garage.

I place as many yummy goods in front of Joy for dinner as I can muster. No interest. The only destination of desire is her bedroom. Once the two of us are cuddled up and comfortable, Joy turns towards my side and takes my hand. She looks at me and proceeds to lock her eyes deep onto mine, which I reciprocate. On and off she slumbers with her eyes half-open or not quite closed. When she awakens fully, rather startled, I talk to her like a mother and daughter would do. "All is well, Joy. Everything will be all right. Your family and friends love you." This lasts past midnight.

Frankly, I again believe her departure is nearing. Disengaging is not an option. We are connected. Again, this is a sleepless night for me. Not so with Joy for she is the one who does the moaning and groaning.

My husband has mentioned before that we should just rent a bed. This is today's mission. This is exactly what I shall do. Fantastic. I am expecting its arrival tomorrow. It's incredible for now I have the meds as well as a fully automated hospital bed rented by the month.

Joy gets up in the morning and eats a good breakfast. Unfortunately, not by her own volition. She can hardly wait to go back to bed. I had plans to take her out to dinner but change my mind. Perhaps tomorrow would be a better day. Just the thought of getting her dressed and into a restaurant seems the opposite of what I believe she is comfortable with at this critical time of her life.

I have predicted her transition for too long, without any backup whatsoever. No more of my earned wisdom. Joy has surprised us numerous times and maybe still has no intention of doing otherwise.

Joy falls again. She still looks pretty banged up when I return from a brief vacation. According to the medical exams, she did not sustain any fractures but keeps crying out at certain movements. She is also compacted in her abdomen for she has not been able to have a bowel movement in four days. Oh, dear!

I immediately run to the store to buy some Activia yogurt and a bag of organic apples. What works for me works for Joy, at least in this department. Then I googled a colonic clinic and off we go. The visit is successful. I wash Joy as much as I can while undressing her and bag every item for the cleaner. Into bed is all this poor woman needs.

As an appetizer at dinnertime, we each eat half an apple. Sautéed zucchinis and a filet follow as the main course, completed by the yogurt and some stool softener. No bread, no rice, no pasta, no potatoes. Not ever her beloved bananas remain on the present menu. This is a serious matter, laced with a bit of humor. Joy gets it, which is the cool part about her. I keep reiterating her condition, what needs to be done, and she does it. When she gives me her long look, I reassure her with, "Just do it, Joy," while nodding my head.

We are a team. She always tells me that she is so glad I am her 'partner.' I do not want to hear those words for at times being her partner is not my desire. As the years go by, my mind has plenty of opportunity to expand. Now, I am her partner.

As time moves on, it is becoming more and more difficult to take care of Joy. Almost every week I am close to making the decision to leave, but then I don't. One voice inside keeps telling me that I am not a nurse and what I am doing is contradicting with my inner being and desire to write. The other voice keeps gently nudging me along, so I stay.

The following day is quite successful. Joy has a bowel movement in the morning, another in the afternoon, and one at night. It worked! I am telling you — eat apples and yogurt. Those combined make and keep you well.

Joy receives her first yogurt early in the morning. Then at breakfast time, I start her off with some apple slices. Nothing else is on her plate at that point, for then she chooses. Am I regimenting her? Yes, I suppose I am, not to give her discomfort, but rather to help her feel more comfortable. Once the apple is eaten, course two arrives — one super fresh laid farm egg, prepared over easy, literally glowing out of the frying pan in the most beautiful orange color one can imagine, laced with a few slices of turkey bacon. A piece of pumpernickel on the side and a smile from her server turns it into a feast for a queen. The third course is more or less a reward called applesauce. She loves it.

A week later, I am in shock at Joy's condition. She does smile upon my arrival. That is all I receive from her during the twenty-four hours. The physical therapist gives her a good workout, which I do realize tires her. Back to bed until I wake her up at four PM with early dinner or late lunch. Joy falls asleep in her chair while eating and I shake her gently to keep her coherent and chewing. What a sight to see. Now what?

Rather than the bedroom, I opt for Joy's car. I quickly collect the necessary goods and we take off for a ride up the coast along the Pacific Ocean. Once at our destination, I take a walk at the harbor, which is completely engulfed in gray. Fog follows us everywhere we turn. Joy sleeps through it all. My conversing, which she normally enjoys, does not find an ear. Daylight savings time adds to our experience. Back in her home, Joy goes right to the table. She has to be hungry. I had formulated a menu from the refrigerator while driving in the car and prepare dinner within minutes of our arrival. Off to bed with Joy and out like a light she goes. Unbelievable.

She opens and closes her eyes to assure herself of my presence. She has not spoken all day and looks mostly down while sitting. She seems so disconnected I feel sad.

The next day is not much better. Once in a while, there is a glimpse of awareness, if only for a moment. I almost feel like celebrating when that happens. That evening we go out to dinner. She just sits there without emotion or any attempt to eat. Suddenly, Joy takes her fork and starts to consume what once was her favorite meal. All right! That is what I like to see. Madame has returned, even if only for a few minutes. Just as suddenly as she appears, she is gone again. We have to take what we can get. Good night dear woman.

The physical therapist visits two to three times a week. I am not really keen on exercising Joy but I also can see her getting weaker if we don't make her move. We walk on a daily basis just before we enter the car to go for a ride. It works.

On the first and second day, Joy produced no bowel movement. Time to administer some stool softener. Most people do not like to talk about this subject, much less read about it, but here we are. Then it happens. Big accident. Whatever you feel like imagining happened. Eventually, this also passes. Thank goodness a diversion occurred. Joy's sister and niece are on the way to visit. Day four is spent socializing and having a good time. Joy's sister insists on taking us all out for dinner. Great Japanese restaurant. Delicious.

It is a week later. Joy looks haggard. She is eating well but not having plenty of fresh air, combined with her ailment, is slowly taking its toll.

Again, I hear that she has not had a bowel movement and has been given two stool softeners and a laxative. Frankly, I am a bit miffed about this kind of news. Nevertheless, the meds were administered and not much else for me to do but be on the alert. After the first success, we get ready for a ride. I decide not to go out for dinner so leave Joy in her pajamas and cover her with a fur-lined leather coat. We cruise along the coast while I stop here and there to take care of some errands.

Back in the car, I smell it. Oh, my goodness. Whatever I envisioned is not a pretty situation. I quickly change my thinking to a better outcome. It is what it is. The leather coat she is wearing might not be so happy but the sheepskin car seat could still be smelling like a rose.

Out of the car and into the house. My hand is resting on Joy's back, pushing her along for she loves to take baby steps with a pause in between. I literally pray to make it to the toilet without losing anything on her thick white carpet. Just enough time to throw a disposable mat under her and there we are. What am I grateful for? The shower. How lucky can we be?

I have mentioned before the importance of being grateful. While learning to give thanks on a constant basis, I am confronted as well with situations I do not want to handle. But I do, partly for what I am, the other part for "I have to do it."

Any idea how strong this makes me? Here we go again. Thank you, thank you. I can do anything coming my way. No problema. Now I can choose. "Do I want to, do I not?" The feeling is grand.

It is night and I put Joy into her hospital bed and go back to the kitchen to clean up. Would you believe, she comes around the corner, letting me know how much she does not like to be alone. My mouth falls open and stays that way. I had forgotten to put up the railing!

How she moans and groans when I ask her to get up. Most certainly I assist her, convinced she needs my help. Apparently not! She is strong willed and probably still convinced inside that she can do anything that crosses her mind.

Joy slumbers for at least an hour. About eleven PM I turn off the light. Almost immediately she goes into action trying to climb out of bed. I brought earplugs over a year ago and have not used them as yet. This would be the moment. While I crawl under the covers, my ears stay sharp for I am curious as to how long it will take her to give up. I hear her legs and arms striking the railing and then, in an instant, she falls back onto her bed, pulls the blankets over her body, and does not make another sound. This hospital bed is a godsend. Those nights were terrible when Joy got up ten or more times.

Two steps Joy makes in the morning without me watching her back and already she is hanging on only one leg while clinging to one side of her walker. Most of the time she picks it up into the air rather than using it for support. What a sight to see. All is well.

Why did I choose the title of this chapter? Yes, I was absolutely sure Joy was saying good bye to us in many different ways!

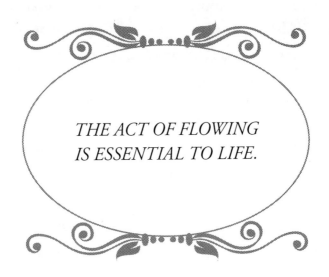

THE ACT OF FLOWING
IS ESSENTIAL TO LIFE.

Time to Move On

Good-bye Joy; good-bye job; good-bye room;
good-bye everything else; good-bye; good-bye.

I have finished journaling. I instinctively know in my heart that this position will come to an end with the completion of my manuscript. Thank you for that.

Thank you for all and everything. The six years together have shaped part of me and for the better. Like all experiences — positive or not — I had the opportunity to draw from this one.

The phone call came. My position has ended. All I feel is relief and gratitude.

The Book of Joy

Joy since has past on.

My time has shifted into a different direction. I have learned and experienced the long and rather difficult road of an Alzheimer Patient, with its depression periods, and the resigning to the present moment, if that.

When your consciousness deceives you and the recognition of family and friends has left the mind, a moment of joy is all we as helpers are able to give.

I spent more than five years with Joy. This time has taught me so much insight and

Unconditional love for humanity. I shall be forever grateful.

May you all be blessed

\# \# \#

Printed in the United States
By Bookmasters